New Treatments in Noninfectious Uveitis

Developments in Ophthalmology

Vol. 51

Series Editor

F. Bandello Milan

New Treatments in Noninfectious Uveitis

Volume Editors

Elisabetta Miserocchi Milan

Giulio Modorati Milan

C. Stephen Foster Cambridge, Mass.

14 figures, 8 in color, and 24 tables, 2012

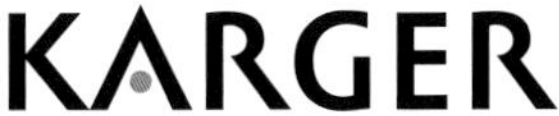

Basel · Freiburg · Paris · London · New York · New Delhi · Bangkok · Beijing · Tokyo · Kuala Lumpur · Singapore · Sydney

Elisabetta Miserocchi
Ocular Immunology and Uveitis Service
Department of Ophthalmology and
Visual Sciences
Scientific Institute San Raffaele
University Vita-Salute
Via Olgettina 60
IT–20132 Milan (Italy)

Giulio Modorati
Ocular Immunology and Uveitis Service
Department of Ophthalmology and
Visual Sciences
Scientific Institute San Raffaele
University Vita-Salute
Via Olgettina 60
IT–20132 Milan (Italy)

C. Stephen Foster
Massachusetts Eye Research and Surgery
Institution
Ocular Immunology and Uveitis Foundation
5 Cambridge Center, 8th Floor
Cambridge, MA 02142 (USA)

This book was generously supported by 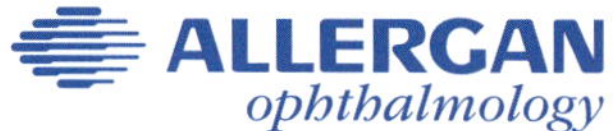

Library of Congress Cataloging-in-Publication Data

New treatments in noninfectious uveitis / volume editors, Elisabetta Miserocchi, Giulio Modorati, C. Stephen Foster.
p. ; cm. -- (Developments in ophthalmology, ISSN 0250-3751 ; v. 51)
Includes bibliographical references and index.
ISBN 978-3-8055-9986-3 (hard cover : alk. paper) -- ISBN 978-3-8055-9987-0 (e-ISBN)
I. Miserocchi, Elisabetta. II. Modorati, Giulio. III. Foster, C. Stephen (Charles Stephen), 1942- IV. Series: Developments in ophthalmology ; v. 51. 0250-3751
[DNLM: 1. Uveitis--drug therapy. W1 DE998NG v.51 2012 / WW 240]

617.7'2--dc23

2012004581

Bibliographic Indices. This publication is listed in bibliographic services, including Current Contents® and Index Medicus.

www.karger.com
Printed in Germany on acid-free and non-aging paper (ISO 9706) by Kraft Druck GmbH, Ettlingen
ISSN 0250–3751
e-ISSN 1662–2790
ISBN 978–3–8055–9986–3
e-ISBN 978–3–8055–9987–0

Contents

List of Contributors

Owhofasa Agbedia
Retinal Imaging Research and Reading Center
Wilmer Eye Institute
Johns Hopkins University School of Medicine
600 North Wolfe Street, Maumenee 745
Baltimore, MD 21287 (USA)
E-Mail oagbedi1@jhmi.edu

Anam Akhlaq
Retinal Imaging Research and Reading Center
Wilmer Eye Institute
Johns Hopkins University School of Medicine
600 North Wolfe Street, Maumenee 745
Baltimore, MD 21287 (USA)
E-Mail anamakhlaq@gmail.com

Abeer Akhtar
Retinal Imaging Research and Reading Center
Wilmer Eye Institute
Johns Hopkins University School of Medicine
600 North Wolfe Street, Maumenee 745
Baltimore, MD 21287 (USA)
E-Mail biya8478@gmail.com

Rachel Annam
Retinal Imaging Research and Reading Center
Wilmer Eye Institute
Johns Hopkins University School of Medicine
600 North Wolfe Street, Maumenee 745
Baltimore, MD 21287 (USA)
E-Mail rannam1@jhmi.edu

Millena Gomes Bittencourt
Retinal Imaging Research and Reading Center
Wilmer Eye Institute
Johns Hopkins University School of Medicine
600 North Wolfe Street, Maumenee 745
Baltimore, MD 21287 (USA)
E-Mail mbitten2@jhmi.edu

Bahram Bodaghi
Department of Ophthalmology
University of Paris VI
Pitié-Salpêtrière Hospital
47 Boulevard de L'Hôpital
FR–75013 Paris (France)
E-Mail bahram.bodaghi@psl.aphp.fr

Marc D. de Smet
Chemin des Allinges 10
CH–1001 Lausanne (Switzerland)
E-Mail mddesmet1@mac.com

Christoph Deuter
Centre for Ophthalmology
University of Tübingen
Schleichstrasse 12–16
DE–72076 Tübingen (Germany)
E-Mail christoph.deuter@med.uni-tuebingen.de

Diana V. Do
Retinal Imaging Research and Reading Center
Wilmer Eye Institute
Johns Hopkins University School of Medicine
600 North Wolfe Street, Maumenee 745
Baltimore, MD 21287 (USA)
E-Mail ddo@jhmi.edu

C. Stephen Foster
Massachusetts Eye Research and Surgery Institution
Ocular Immunology and Uveitis Foundation
5 Cambridge Center, 8th Floor
Cambridge, MA 02142 (USA)
E-Mail sfoster@mersi.com

Julie Gueudry
Department of Ophthalmology
Charles Nicolle University Hospital
1 rue de Germont
FR–76031 Rouen (France)
E-Mail julie.gueudry@chu-rouen.fr

Arnd Heiligenhaus
Department of Ophthalmology
St. Franziskus Hospital
Hohenzollernring 74
DE–48145 Münster (Germany)
E-Mail arnd.heiligenhaus@uveitis-zentrum.de

Maren Hennig
Department of Ophthalmology
St. Franziskus Hospital
Hohenzollernring 74
DE–48145 Münster (Germany)
E-Mail maren.hennig@uveitis-zentrum.de

Mohamed Ibrahim
Retinal Imaging Research and Reading Center
Wilmer Eye Institute
Johns Hopkins University School of Medicine
600 North Wolfe Street, Maumenee 745
Baltimore, MD 21287 (USA)
E-Mail mibrahi5@jhmi.edu

Dino D. Klisovic
Midwest Retina
6655 Post Road
Dublin, OH 43016 (USA)
E-Mail dklisov@yahoo.com

Jonathan Kruh
Massachusetts Eye Research and Surgery Institution
Ocular Immunology and Uveitis Foundation
5 Cambridge Center, 8th Floor
Cambridge, MA 02142 (USA)
E-Mail jkruh@mersi.com

Phuc LeHoang
Department of Ophthalmology
University of Paris VI
Pitié-Salpêtrière Hospital
83 Boulevard de L'Hôpital
FR–75013 Paris (France)
E-Mail phuc.lehoang@psl.ap-hop-paris.fr

Sue Lightman
UCL Institute of Ophthalmology
Moorfields Eye Hospital
162 City Road
London EC1V 2PD (UK)
E-Mail s.lightman@ucl.ac.uk

Hongting Liu
Retinal Imaging Research and Reading Center
Wilmer Eye Institute
Johns Hopkins University School of Medicine
600 North Wolfe Street, Maumenee 745
Baltimore, MD 21287 (USA)
E-Mail hliu43@jhmi.edu

Elisabetta Miserocchi
Ocular Immunology and Uveitis Service
Department of Ophthalmology and Visual Sciences
Scientific Institute San Raffaele
University Vita-Salute
Via Olgettina 60
IT–20132 Milan (Italy)
E-Mail miserocchi.elisabetta@hsr.it

Giulio Modorati
Ocular Immunology and Uveitis Service
Department of Ophthalmology and Visual Sciences
Scientific Institute San Raffaele
University Vita-Salute
Via Olgettina 60
IT–20132 Milan (Italy)
E-Mail modorati.giulio@hsr.it

Burkhard Möller
Department of Rheumatology, Allergology and Immunology
Inselspital
University of Bern
CH–3010 Bern (Switzerland)
E-Mail burkhard.moeller@insel.ch

Quan Dong Nguyen
Retinal Imaging Research and Reading Center
Wilmer Eye Institute
Johns Hopkins University School of Medicine
600 North Wolfe Street, Maumenee 745
Baltimore, MD 21287 (USA)
E-Mail qnguyen4@jhmi.edu

Yasir Jamal Sepah
Retinal Imaging Research and Reading Center
Wilmer Eye Institute
Johns Hopkins University School of Medicine
600 North Wolfe Street, Maumenee 745
Baltimore, MD 21287 (USA)
E-Mail ysepah2@jhmi.edu

Nicole Stübiger
Department of Ophthalmology
Campus Benjamin Franklin
Charité
Universitätsmedizin Berlin
Hindenburgdamm 30
DE–12203 Berlin (Germany)
E-Mail nicole.stuebiger@charite.de

Christoph Tappeiner
Department of Ophthalmology
Inselspital
University of Bern
CH–3010 Bern (Switzerland)
E-Mail christoph.tappeiner@insel.ch

Simon R.J. Taylor
UCL Institute of Ophthalmology
Moorfields Eye Hospital
162 City Road
London EC1V 2PD (UK)
E-Mail s.r.taylor@ucl.ac.uk

Oren Tomkins-Netzer
UCL Institute of Ophthalmology
Moorfields Eye Hospital
162 City Road
London EC1V 2PD (UK)
E-Mail oren.tomkins@gmail.com

Manfred Zierhut
Centre for Ophthalmology
University of Tübingen
Schleichstrasse 12–16
DE–72076 Tübingen (Germany)
E-Mail manfred.zierhut@med.uni-tuebingen.de

Preface

Uveitis is a potentially blinding inflammatory disease that presents a therapeutic challenge for the general ophthalmologist and even for the uveitis specialist. The importance of this sight-threatening disease is translated into numbers, with important studies demonstrating that uveitis is the cause of 2.8–10% of all cases of blindness.

The primary goal of therapy in patients with uveitis should be controlling intraocular inflammation, reducing the risk of ocular complications and secondary visual loss. However, when we are faced with severe inflammatory ocular disease, we always have to balance the risk and benefit of preserving vision versus the occurrence of potentially severe treatment-related adverse events.

The dawn of the modern age for the treatment of uveitis came in 1950, with the employment of corticosteroids that have completely revolutionized the treatment of ocular inflammatory disease. But, with the increasing use of corticosteroids over time and the discovery of exciting results both for patients and physicians in treating uveitis, the long-term adverse events of corticosteroids become rapidly evident. It became clear that corticosteroids were potent and excellent drugs to control autoimmune uveitis, leading to rapid resolution of intraocular inflammation, but their safety profile and the secondary occurrence of systemic side effects render their use a double-edged sword.

Due to the high morbidity related to long-term treatment with corticosteroids, physicians were stimulated to find corticosteroid-sparing therapeutic agents, such as the chemotherapeutic agents.

Most of the systemic immunomodulatory drugs employed in ophthalmology have been adopted from other specialties, such as rheumatology and dermatology.

The new era of corticosteroid-sparing drugs created a 'new therapeutic philosophy' in the management of intraocular inflammation among uveitis specialists around the world. The first generation of immunosuppressive agents employed in uveitis were the alkylating agents in the early 1950s , followed by the antimetabolites methotrexate and azathioprine in the 1960s and cyclosporin A in the 1970s. Cyclosporin A has remained one of the only immunosuppressants prescribed on-label for ocular immune-mediated disorders.

Better understanding of the immune system and inflammatory pathways were further discovered between the 1980s and the 1990s. During this period, the interactions between specific cytokines and cell surface receptors led to the development of novel therapeutic approaches.

The great revolution in the treatment of uveitis came in the 1990s with the introduction of the so-called 'new therapeutic agents', known as a biologic response modifiers. These agents, created through modern bioengineering techniques, were designed to act as cell-specific immunosuppressants by the direct inhibition of cytokines or cell surface molecules. This would allow for more precise modulation of the immune system without having the effects of a systemic and global immune suppression.

During the last decade, an increasing number of new drugs have been introduced in the field of rheumatology for the treatment of autoimmune diseases, such as rheumatoid arthritis, and have been subsequently explored in the treatment of uveitis patients with exciting results.

The therapeutic armamentarium of the uveitis specialist has expanded enormously compared to previous generations. New randomized clinical trials are investigating the use of new treatment options for ocular inflammatory diseases.

The desire to avoid systemic side effects from corticosteroids and immunosuppressants has driven the continuing search for effective agents with an improved safety profile, but also the increasing use of local drug administration, which can avoid systemic side effects.

For this reason, the development of intraocular therapy has generated an increasing interest in the last decade as an alternative treatment to control ocular inflammatory diseases and inflammatory macular edema, which is the most important cause of visual loss in patients with uveitis.

Intraocular implants which release corticosteroids for a prolonged period within the vitreous cavity have been recently developed for treating ocular inflammation. The first implant designed was a nonerodible implant device that released fluocinolone acetonide, while the one most recently introduced on the market is the bioerodible polymer that releases dexamethasone. In clinical trials, both implants have been shown to be effective in reducing intraocular inflammation in patients with intermediate or posterior uveitis. Certain clinical situations, particularly with asymmetric uveitis or severe inflammatory macular edema, may in fact favor intravitreal treatment over systemic treatment. Short-term intravitreal therapy can be employed as well, with intravitreal corticosteroid or methotrexate injections.

Patients with uveitis and ocular inflammatory diseases are in desperate need of effective therapeutic agents which cannot only eliminate inflammation and prevent recurrences but also protect the patients from potential side effects. In addition, we believe that all currently available drugs should be approved by the regulatory bodies as soon as possible so that they can be of benefit to all patients.

Today, the horizon of uveitis treatment appears very bright compared to a decade ago given the many therapeutic agents and approaches for uveitis and ocular inflammatory diseases. Different classes of new agents, delivery systems and novel methods of safe and effective administration of pharmacologic agents are under investigation. Hopefully, in the near future such efforts will lead to an increasing number of therapeutic options for our patients that will improve not only the vision but also the quality of life of these patients.

This book was designed to bring together the principles of therapy of patients with noninfectious uveitis and the most recent therapeutic options that can be offered to the patient. Its aim is to help educate residents, update general ophthalmologists and uveitis specialists on the latest innovative treatment options for patients who have noninfectious uveitis. After an outline of the treatment principles and the most conventional treatment options, the book covers a large number of topics on the newer available agents for intraocular inflammation.

The authors bring together their personal experience and full teaching acumen to each chapter, culminating in a single book that brings to the forefront the importance of the challenge in the treatment of uveitis. We hope that each chapter will stimulate the interest of readers working in this particular field of uveitis.

Elisabetta Miserocchi, Milan
Giulio Modorati, Milan
C. Stephen Foster, Cambridge, Mass.

Miserocchi E, Modorati G, Foster CS (eds): New Treatments in Noninfectious Uveitis.
Dev Ophthalmol. Basel, Karger, 2012, vol 51, pp 1–6

The Philosophy of Treatment of Uveitis: Past, Present and Future

Jonathan Kruh · C. Stephen Foster

Massachusetts Eye Research and Surgery Institution, Ocular Immunology and Uveitis Foundation, Cambridge, Mass., USA

Abstract

Treatment of inflammatory diseases of the eye is especially challenging. Although physicians in antiquity had recognized the existence of ocular inflammatory disease, their lack of understanding of the immune system made successful treatment almost impossible. Throughout the 20th century, great advances in the diagnosis and treatment of uveitis led to unique treatment options. The development of corticosteroids in 1949 and its application to the eye in 1950 revolutionized therapeutic strategies. As the use of corticosteroids became more prevalent in treating ocular inflammatory diseases, so did its side effects. Due to the high morbidity in conjunction with long-term corticosteroid use, physicians pursued other agents, specifically through the employment of chemotherapeutic agents. The shift from exclusive corticosteroid monotherapy to steroid-sparing immunomodulatory therapy reshaped the landscape of treating ocular inflammatory disease. Over time, with increased efforts, new therapies were studied, trialed, and brought to the market. Today, in comparison to any other time in history, physicians have available to them the largest array of effective agents for achieving the ultimate goal: corticosteroid-free, durable remission.

The earliest recorded documentation of uveitis dates back to ancient Egyptian times, via accounts found on the Edwin Smith surgical papyrus, now housed in the library of the New York Academy of Medicine [1]. The writings date back to 1700 BC, but include references to concepts from earlier periods in ancient Egypt dating back to 2640 BC. Physicians with specific focus on the eye are known to have existed at least back to the 6th Egyptian Dynasty (2400 BC). The Royal Oculist, Pepi-Ankh-Or-Iri, is noted on ancient markings near the tomb of the Great Pyramid of Cheops. He was the physician to the Pharaoh and bared the title 'palace eye physician', as well as 'guardian of the anus'. Although in modern times, these two titles appear to be disparate toward one another, this was not always the case. Since ancient times, cleansing the body of toxic elements, known as 'purgative therapy', had been utilized as the standard treatment for many different diseases.

Further treatment modalities came to light in the Ebers papyrus [2, 3]. This document addressed multiple different ocular diseases and their treatment. Although many of the treatments outlined in the Ebers papyrus are now regarded as primitive and ineffective, there are a few which have a sound basis. Of the 237 medication recipes, 100 were detailed for the treatment of ocular disease. Included were medications to be used for miosis and mydriasis.

Until the late 18th and early 19th century, few advances were made in ocular care. In 1830, MacKenzie wrote a text for the treatment of eye disease. In addition to bloodletting, purging, and blistering therapy, some novel concepts were added [4]. These included: dilation of the pupil with tincture of belladonna and the use of antimony, nauseants, and opiates for pain relief.

In the early 20th century, fever therapy became a novel approach to the treatment of old problems. Fever therapy was induced by intramuscular injection of milk or intravenous administration of triple typhoid H antigen. The goal of this therapy was to raise one's core body temperature to ~40°C. It was postulated that the efficacy of heat therapy is secondary to the endogenous release of corticosteroids in the body during these periods of high stress. Although at times this therapy was successful, it was often unpredictable and sometimes even deadly.

The dawn of the modern age for the treatment of uveitis came shortly thereafter, in 1950, with the employment of corticosteroid for treating uveitis. From the time of its inception by Gordon [5], it was clear that it was going to be a major advance in the field of ocular inflammation. For many patients with inflammatory disorders, this discovery appeared to them as a light at the end of a dark tunnel. Both physicians and patients alike embraced the usage of this agent, despite its potential for long-term adverse effects. As the years progressed, the side effects of chronic corticosteroid use became widely observed and published. Some of the secondary systemic effects that became evident were electrolyte imbalances, myopathy, osteoporosis, aseptic necrosis of the humeral and femoral heads, tendon rupture, nausea, peptic ulcer, bowel perforation, pancreatitis, poor wound healing, easy bruising neurological disturbances, menstrual irregularities, Cushingoid state, diabetes, hirsutism, suppression of adrenocortical pituitary axis, growth suppression, weight gain, and thromboembolism [6–11]. Ocular effects included an increased incidence for the development of cataracts, glaucoma, central serous retinopathy, and activation of herpes simplex virus [7, 11, 12].

Although chronic corticosteroid use suppressed many inflammatory diseases, most reasonable physicians felt that the side effect profile of prolonged corticosteroid use placed upon the patient was unacceptable. Therefore, corticosteroid-sparing immunomodulatory agents were developed. Soon thereafter, the first generation of immunosuppressive agents were investigated for their efficacy in treating uveitis.

The first group developed were the alkylating agents, mainly cyclophosphamide and chlorambucil. Their main action is the inhibition of lymphoid proliferation. Cyclophosphamide's emergence into the medical world did not occur until the 1950s.

Its parent molecule, nitrogen mustard, was originally designed for chemical warfare during World War I. Its therapeutic efficacy lies in its ability to suppress the bone marrow, causing leukopenia and aplasia of lymphoid tissue [13]. Its first reported use in the 1950s was for the treatment of uveitis by Roda-Perez [14–16].

Chlorambucil, created in the 1950s, was originally used for the treatment of malignant lymphoma [14]. Its first reported use in the ophthalmic world was in 1970, when Mamo and Azzam utilized the drug for the treatment of the uveitis associated with Adamantiades-Behçet's disease [17].

During this same time period, another category of immunosuppressive agents were being investigated. The antimetabolites function through inhibition of key enzymatic reactions necessary for cell reproduction. The original antimetabolites created were methotrexate and azathioprine. Although methotrexate was discovered in 1948, it took almost 20 years before it made its way into the ophthalmic world. Originally, this drug was used for the treatment of acute leukemia in children [18]. By 1965, the first reports for use in the treatment of ocular inflammatory disorders began to emerge by Wong and Hersh [19]. Azathioprine was brought onto the market in the 1960s, originally developed for the use of immunosuppression in transplant patients, and in the treatment of autoimmune diseases [20]. By 1966, Newell began using it to treat ocular immune-mediated disorders [21, 22].

It was not until the 1970s when noncytotoxic immunosuppressives first made their appearance in the treatment of autoimmune disease. In the early 1970s, cyclosporin A (CSA) was derived from cultures of the fungi *Tolypocladium inflatum* [23]. The effectiveness of CSA for the treatment of autoimmune uveitis was first reported by Nussenblatt et al. [24, 25] in 1983. Significant nephrotoxicity and systemic hypertension led to additional investigation into future therapies. Tacrolimus was discovered in 1984 from a strain of fungi in the soil, *Streptomyces tsukubaensis* [26]. Shortly thereafter in the 1990s, Sirolimus was isolated from the strain of fungi *Streptomyces hygroscopicus* [27]. The next generation of antimetabolite therapy was mycophenolate mofetil. It arrived onto the scene in 1995, originally approved for the prevention of solid organ transplant rejection. Shortly thereafter, it was employed by uveitis specialists for treating patients with unremitting uveitis.

Throughout the 1980s and 1990s, the particulars of the immune system and inflammatory pathways were further elucidated. With a greater understanding of the interactions between specific cytokines and cell surface receptors, novel approaches for new treatments were created. As the 1990s progressed, there emerged a new series of drugs known as biologic response modifiers. These agents were created through biology techniques, as opposed to pure chemistry. It was theorized that through the inhibition of unique cytokines or cell surface receptors there could be cell-specific targeting of immunosuppression. This would allow for more precise modulation of the immune system without global suppression.

Murmonab (Orthoclone OKT3®) was the first of its kind in this class; it was developed by Ortho Pharmaceuticals in the mid-1980s. It was used to treat acute, glucocorticoid-resistant rejection of allogenic renal transplants [28]. The next wave of drugs came in the late 1990s. These drugs were designed with the intent of treating specific autoimmune disorders, in particular rheumatoid arthritis, Crohn's disease, and inflammatory bowel disease. One of the first of these to be manufactured was etanercept (Enbrel®); it was originally approved in 1999 for the treatment of rheumatoid arthritis. It is composed of soluble tumor necrosis factor (TNF) receptor and human IgG Fc fragment. Soon after, many new biologics appeared on the market, some of which included abatacept (Orencia®, target: B7), adalimumab (Humira®, target: TNF-α), daclizumab (Zenapax®, target: CD25), infliximab (Remicade®, target: TNF-α), anakinra (Kinaret®, target: IL-1 receptor), rituximab (Rituxa®, target: CD20), and tocilizumab (Actemra®, target: IL-6 receptor). In addition, two other treatment modalities of interest developed were intravenous immunoglobulin and interferon-γ.

As compared with previous generations, we are in a unique position with regard to the treatment of ocular inflammatory diseases. Today, there are a large variety of drugs in our armamentarium that we can use to treat, as well as to actually cure inflammatory disease. That being said, it is imperative that it is understood that the goal of treatment for every patient with ocular inflammation is to achieve corticosteroid-free durable remission.

We suggest a stepladder algorithmic approach for the treatment of noninfectious uveitis. The process in deciding which medication to start a patient on is based upon a multitude of factors. Some of these factors include age, sex, social history, past medical history, compliance factors, and, most importantly, their specific ocular inflammatory disease. The administration of these medications and the monitoring of these patients becomes a joint effort between the ophthalmologist and multiple sub-specialists (rheumatology, oncology, and hematology).

The first step for most patients with ocular inflammation begins with the initiation of corticosteroid treatment; this may be dispensed topically, through local injection, or systemically. Corticosteroids are often started because they usually are able to control inflammation quickly. Although excellent at quelling inflammation initially, oftentimes these agents are not curative for the problem but rather function as a 'band-aid' remedy. Many times, this patient population is unable to completely wean off corticosteroid therapy without having a recurrence of their uveitis.

These corticosteroid-dependent patients must then move forward with a plan for alternative long-term therapy; again, the primary goal is for the patient to be in remission, off all corticosteroids. Ultimately if this is achieved, these patients are afforded a much more favorable long-term outcome, free of the devastating effects of chronic corticosteroid use.

The next step in the stepladder paradigm is the use of nonsteroidal anti-inflammatory drugs (NSAIDs). NSAID therapy includes some commonly known drugs, e.g. Celebrex®, Ibuprofen, and Naprosyn. Treatment with these drugs requires blood monitoring of kidney and liver function, as well as, in some patients, gastrointestinal prophylaxis with a proton pump inhibitor or a histamine H2 receptor antagonist. If the patient continues to have chronic or recurrent active inflammation, a more aggressive approach to their problem must be undertaken. Such patients require immunomodulatory therapy with chemotherapeutic agents. The emotional transition to the induction of chemotherapy for most patients, as well as for many physicians, can be the most formidable challenge to the achievement of corticosteroid-free durable remission.

The choice of chemotherapeutics is case-specific and escalates in a stepwise approach. The drug chosen should offer the most favorable side effect profile and efficacy for the patients' specific ocular inflammatory disease. Once initiated, the patient must be consistently monitored to safeguard against toxicity and intolerable side effects. As needed, it may be necessary to titrate their dosage, add a second or a third agent, or discontinue the drug altogether, if not tolerated or found not to be therapeutic. For less aggressive forms of uveitis, often the decision might be to pick a medication that can be taken orally, e.g. methotrexate, mycophenolate mofetil, or cyclosporin. For more recalcitrant forms of inflammatory disease, the choice may be to add an adjunct medication given either subcutaneously (e.g. adalimumab), or via infusion therapy. (e.g. infliximab and cyclophosphamide). It must be reiterated that there is never room to allow for undue side effects whether it be life threatening, e.g. leukopenia, or quality of life threatening, e.g. nausea and fatigue.

Thus, the treatment of uveitis entails not only having a comprehensive knowledge base on the treatment patterns of specific uveitic entities, but an art in the prescribing of medication. There are many different 'cocktails' of therapy one might craft with the different drugs via dosage titration and administration. Furthermore, it may become necessary for the addition of surgical intervention to the treatment plan. At times, this may be essential in not only quieting the eye but also in achieving better vision. Ultimately, it is our recommendation that there should be no reduction of treatment until the patient has remained in remission, off all corticosteroids, for at a minimum of 2 years. At that time, one may attempt to slowly taper the dosage of medication and/or the treatment intervals. It is only after achieving 2 years of quiescence of all corticosteroids which we feel that the patient has the best chance of remaining in remission and possibly cured of his/her disease.

As we look ahead, the future for the treatment of ocular inflammatory disease has never been brighter. There is great hope that there will be continued advances in the development of novel medications. Immunomodulating therapies will become increasingly more sensitive in the targeting of specific mediators that regulate inflammation. Patients will continue to have improved outcomes while experiencing fewer toxicities from their medications. The goal still remains the same: long-lasting, corticosteroid-free, durable remission.

References

1 Breasted J: The Edwin Smith Surgical Papyrus. Chicago, University of Chicago Press, 1930.
2 Ebbell B: Die altagyptische Chirurgie. Die chirurgischen Abschnitte des Papyrus E. Smith and Papyrus Ebers. Oslo, Dybwad, 1939.
3 Hirschberg J: The History of Ophthalmology, vol 1 Antiquity. Bonn, Wayenborgh, 1982.
4 MacKenzie W: A Practical Treatise on the Diseases of the Eye. London, Longman, Rees, Orme, Brown & Green, 1830, pp 422–457.
5 Gordon D: Prednisone and prednisolone in ocular inflammatory disease. Am J Ophthalmol 1956;41:593–600.
6 Fujikawa L, Meisler D, Novik R: Hyperosmolar hyperglycemic nonkeotic coma. A complication of short-term systemic corticosteroids. Ophthalmology 1983;90:1239–1242.
7 Wakakura M, Ishikawa S: Central serous chorioretinopathy complicating systemic corticosteroid treatment. Br J Ophthalmol 1984;68:329–331.
8 Polito C, La Manna A, Papale MR: Delayed pubertal growth spurt and normal adult height attainment in boys receiving long-term alternate day prednisone therapy. Clin Pediatr 1999;38:279–285.
9 American College of Rheumatology Task Force on Osteoporosis Guidelines. Recommendations for the prevention and treatment of glucocorticoid-induced osteoporosis. Arthritis Rheum 1996;39:1791–1801.
10 Huscher D, Thiele K, Gromnica-Ihle E, Hein G, Demary W, Dreher R, Zink A, Buttgereit F: Dose-related patterns of glucocorticoid-induced side effects. Ann Rheum Dis 2009;68:1119–1124.
11 Nussenblatt R, Whitcup S: Uveitis Fundamentals and Clinical Practice. St Louis, Mosby, 2010, pp 81–84.
12 Pfefferman R, Gombos GM, Kountz SL: Ocular complications after renal transplantation. Ann Ophthalmol 1977;9:467–470.
13 Krumbhaar EB, Krumbhaar HD: The blood and bone marrow in yellow cross gas (mustard gas) poisoning: changes produced in the bone marrow of fatal cases. J Med Res 1919;40:497–507.
14 Gery I, Nussenblatt RB: Immunosuppressive Drugs; in Sears ML (ed.): Pharmacology of the Eye. Berlin, Springer, 1984, pp 586–609.
15 Roda-Perez E: Sobre un case se uveitis de etiologia ignota tratado con mostaza introgenada. Rev Clin Esp 1951;40:265–267.
16 Roda-Perez E: El tratamiento de las uveitis de etiologia ignota con mostaza nitrogenada. Arch Soc Ofial Hisp Am 1952;12:131–151.
17 Mamo JG, Azzam SA: Treatment of Behcet's disease with chlorambucil. Arch Ophthalmol 1970;84:446–450.
18 Farber S, Diamond LK, Mercer RD: Temporary remissions in acute leukemia in children produced by folic antagonist 4-amethopteroylglutamic acid (aminopterin). N Engl J Med 1948;238:787–793.
19 Wong VG, Hersh EM: Methotrexate in the therapy of cyclitis. Trans Am Acad Ophthalmol Otolaryngol 1965;69:279–293.
20 Rapini RP, Jordan RE, Wolverton SE: Cytotoxic agents; in Wolverton SE, Wilkins JK (eds): Systemic Drugs for Skin Diseases. Philadelphia, WB Saunders, 1991, pp 125–151.
21 Newell FW, Krill AE: Treatment of uveitis with azathioprine (Imuran). Trans Ophthalmol Soc UK 1967;87:499–511.
22 Newell FW, Krill AE, Thompson A: The treatment of uveitis with six-mercaptopurine. Am J Ophthalmol 1966;61:1250–1255.
23 Borel JF: The history of cyclosporine A and its significance; in White DJG (ed.): Cyclosporin A. New York, Elsevier Biomedical Press, 1982, pp 5–17.
24 Nussenblatt RB, Palestine AG, Rook AH: Treatment of intraocular inflammation with Cyclosporine A. Lancet 1983;1:235–238.
25 Nussenblatt RB, Palestine AG, Chan CC: Cyclosporine A therapy in the treatment of intraocular inflammatory disease resistant to systemic corticosteroids and cytotoxic agents. Am J Ophthalmol 1983;96:275–282.
26 Kino T, Hatanaka H, Hashimoto M: FK-506, a novel immunosuppressant isolated from Streptomyces. I. Fermentation isolation. Physico-chemical and biological characteristics. J Antibiot 1987;40:1249–1255.
27 Sehgal S, Baker H, Vezina C: Rapamycin (AY-22, 989), a new antifungal antibiotic. II. Fermentation, isolation and characterization. J Antibiot 1975;28:727–732.
28 Ortho Multicenter Transplant Study Group: A randomized clinical trial of OKT3 monoclonal antibody for acute rejection of cadaveric renal transplants. N Engl J Med 1985;313:337–342.

Jonathan Kruh
Massachusetts Eye Research and Surgery Institution
Ocular Immunology and Uveitis Foundation
5 Cambridge Center, 8th Floor
Cambridge, MA 02142 (USA)
Tel. +1 617 621 6377, E-Mail jkruh@mersi.com

Miserocchi E, Modorati G, Foster CS (eds): New Treatments in Noninfectious Uveitis.
Dev Ophthalmol. Basel, Karger, 2012, vol 51, pp 7–28

The Gold Standard of Noninfectious Uveitis: Corticosteroids

Phuc LeHoang

Department of Ophthalmology, University of Paris VI, Pitié-Salpêtrière Hospital, Paris, France

Abstract

Corticosteroids (CS) are considered to be the mainstay of therapy in noninfectious uveitis. They can be administered only after excluding an infectious origin or a possible masquerade syndrome. Different CS preparations can be used with various modes of administration: topical, periocular, intraocular, systemic or a combination of the above routes. Their indications depend upon numerous factors, among them the type (involving or not the posterior segment), the severity, the uni-/bilaterality, the chronicity of the intraocular inflammation. The induction treatment must be aggressive in order to overcome the intraocular inflammation as rapidly as possible avoiding permanent tissue damage. The dosage regimen is then tapered according to the clinical response and after a minimum period of quiescence. The maintenance CS treatment should not exceed 6–12 months under the threat of severe adverse effects. In chronic cases, high-dosage CS monotherapy cannot be used; it is important to add an immunomodulatory treatment on time when a long-term therapy is needed to control the disease. Although CS represent the first line of treatment, the type of clinical response to CS is not a reliable indicator of the effectiveness of immunomodulation: a noninfectious uveitis unresponsive to CS may respond to immunomodulation alone or combined with CS.

In most of the cases, the etiology of noninfectious uveitis is unknown. Despite a specific entity diagnosis, there is no specific treatment available. The main objective is to suppress the inflammatory responses and its consequences by taking nonspecific measures including topical, regional and/or systemic corticosteroids (CS), mydriatics cycloplegics, nonsteroidal anti-inflammatory agents, immunomodulating agents, laser photocoagulation.

CS are considered to be the mainstay of therapy in noninfectious uveitis, although there are no results from randomized clinical trials. The use of CS is based on historical experiences and on the information coming from case series. CS modes of action, effectiveness, limitations, contraindications and adverse effects have been well known for decades. That situation can explain why physicians still currently tend to utilize

CS as the first line drug: they know exactly what they may expect and thus feel more secure as they can prevent most of the milder side effects. They also know that the appearance of severe adverse effects, including bad quality of life, is the major signal for switching to another therapeutic regimen. The effectiveness of CS can be evaluated in the short-term, but it is difficult to estimate how CS may improve the final visual prognosis.

In order to minimize severe intolerance to chronic use of CS, it is advisable to initiate high-dose CS during the acute stage of the disease in order to control the intraocular inflammation as rapidly as possible and then taper progressively the CS to the minimum active threshold dose. If the minimum dosage capable of controlling the inflammation is too high and intolerable for the patient, one should add CS-sparing drugs. In some specific entities, such as Behçet's disease or birdshot chorioretinopathy for example, CS are known to be insufficient at tolerable doses. In such cases, immunomodulatory therapy can be initiated at the onset of the disease.

When May We Use Corticosteroid Therapy in Noninfectious Uveitis?

One must be certain that the uveitis is not due to a direct infectious process. A complete workup must be performed according to the past medical history (including the family history, the sexual history), the clinical symptoms and signs, the general medical condition, the comprehensive ocular examination. Orientated diagnostic testing is informative in atypical presentations. Blood and sometimes ocular fluid samples can confirm the absence of infection whether bacterial, viral, parasitic or fungal before administering high doses of glucocorticoids. If the uveitis is unilateral or is known to have been previously resistant to CS therapy administered elsewhere, one should be very cautious and should not hesitate to repeat an extensive workup (fig. 1). Because of the current tuberculosis resurgence, we always performed a tuberculin skin test and/or a Quantiferon-TB Gold test before initiating an aggressive CS therapy. If the patient is coming from a strongyloidiasis-infected area, a systematic anthelminthic treatment is administered before CS therapy (ivermectin given in a single dose of 200 μg/kg for 1 or 2 days).

One must also rule out a masquerade syndrome mimicking a noninfectious uveitis. Unlike benign conditions such as an intravitreal hemorrhage, ignoring a malignant disease such as a primary intraocular non-Hodgkin lymphoma will have serious consequences. A primary intraocular non-Hodgkin lymphoma must be suspected in an elderly with white painless eyes presenting with a dense vitritis, scarce small deep yellowish retinal infiltrations mainly if the apparent inflammation was known to be poorly responsive to moderate doses of systemic or regional CS in the past. The same caution must be applied in the case of retinoblastoma in childhood or any other malignant disease (leukemia, amelanotic melanomas. . .).

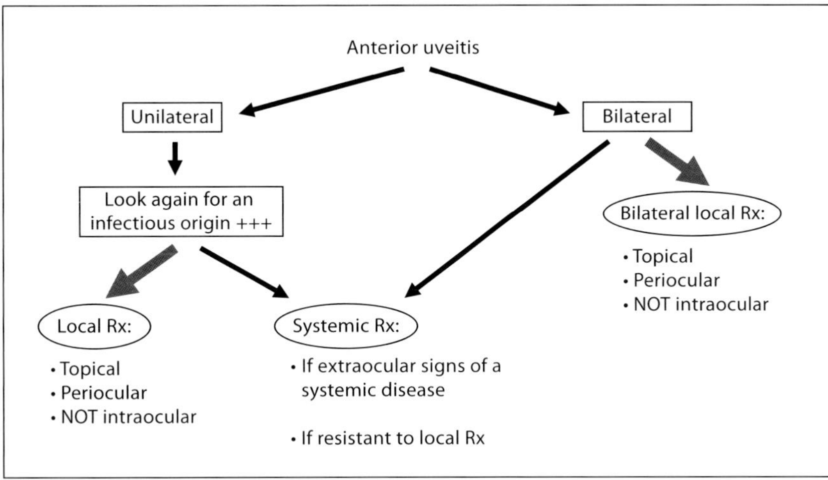

Fig. 1. Corticosteroids: therapeutic strategies (1). Rx = Treatment; TNF = tumor necrosis factor.

Pharmacology

The term CS refers to both glucocorticoids and mineralocorticoids, but is often used as a synonym for glucocorticoids. They are naturally produced by the adrenal cortex. Glucocorticoids can control or prevent inflammation by suppressing the migration of polymorphonuclear leukocytes and fibroblasts and by reversing capillary permeability. They have potent anti-inflammatory and immunosuppressive properties. As a consequence, glucocorticoids are widely used as drugs to treat inflammatory conditions such as arthritis, dermatitis, and noninfectious uveitis and as an adjunct therapy for autoimmune diseases.

Nowadays, only synthetic molecules are used in clinical practice. All CS have 21 carbon atoms, forming a molecule with four rings. Modifications of the basic structure result in compounds with various biologic properties. Thus, their respective anti-inflammatory activity, sodium-retaining activity, duration of action, intraocular pressure (IOP) increase, transcorneal penetration can vary from one molecule to another. The glucocorticoid molecule enters passively the target cell. It then binds to a specific cytoplasmic receptor (glucocorticoid receptor). The cytoplasmic steroid-receptor complex becomes activated, crosses the nuclear membrane and binds to specific sites of the DNA called glucocorticoid response elements. This binding controls the transcription of specific genes promoting or inhibiting the production of certain mRNAs. The rate of protein synthesis of the target cell is thereby modified, activated for some, inhibited for others. These mechanisms explain the rapidity and the multiplicity of action of a single hormone binding to a single receptor. Cells involved in inflammatory reactions are the main targets: lymphocytes, monocytes, local resident cells such as endothelial cells, fibroblasts, hepatocytes. Nuclear translocation of

Table 1. Relative anti-inflammatory activity of glucocorticoids

Drug	Relative anti-inflammatory potency	Systemic equivalent dosages, mg	Half-life, h
Low Potency			
Hydrocortisone	1.0	20	8–12
Cortisone	0.8	25	8–12
Medium Potency			
Prednisone	4.0	5	18–36
Prednisolone	4.0	5	18–36
Methylprednisolone	5.0	4	18–36
Triamcinolone	5.0	4	18–36
High Potency			
Dexamethasone	~25	0.75	36–54
Betamethasone	~25	0.75	36–54

cytoplasmic glucocorticoid receptors has been shown in the iris-ciliary body and the adjacent corneoscleral structure in rabbits. The relative anti-inflammatory activity of glucocorticoids is summarized in table 1 [1].

Preparations and Administration

Topical Preparations and Administration Route

Different CS preparations of variable anti-inflammatory potencies are available for ophthalmic topical use (table 2) [2–4]. The more potent the preparations are, the more ocular side effects are observed (elevated IOP, cataract). Most of them are listed in table 3 in decreasing order of anti-inflammatory potency. Dexamethasone is theoretically the most potent topical steroid. However, the better transcorneal penetration and the higher molar aqueous humor concentration of prednisolone acetate make it theoretically relatively more potent than dexamethasone alcohol/sodium phosphate drops. In rabbits, there are controversial results concerning the corneal and anterior chamber penetration of various CS preparations depending on whether the corneal epithelium is intact or not. Besides the drug concentrations, numerous metabolic parameters can influence the therapeutic effectiveness of different CS preparations: glucocorticoid receptor binding affinity, local enzyme-induced inactivation, intraocular clearance, inherent anti-inflammatory potency. In clinical practice, other factors influencing the effectiveness of topical CS administration should not be overlooked such as the dosage frequency or compliance problems, among which the need for shaking a suspension.

Table 2. Relative anti-inflammatory effects and peak aqueous concentration of topical CS preparations (drops)

Drug	Relative anti-inflammatory potency	Peak aqueous concentration ng/ml	Peak molar anterior chamber concentration 10^{-9} mol/ml	Relative anti-inflammatory effect
Prednisolone acetate 1%	1.0	670	1.66	32
Prednisolone sodium phosphate 0.5%	1.0	26	0.053	1
Dexamethasone alcohol 0.1%	6.25	31	0.079	9
Betamethasone sodium phosphate 0.5%	6.25	8	0.015	2

Table 3. Topical CS preparations: in descending order of intraocular anti-inflammatory potency

Drug	Concentration, %	Formulation
Dexamethasone alcohol	0.1	suspension
	0.05	ointment
Dexamethasone sodium phosphate	0.1	solution
	0.05	ointment
Prednisolone acetate	0.12–0.125–1.0	suspension
Prednisolone sodium phosphate	0.12–0.5–1.0	solution
Prednisolone phosphate	0.25	ointment
Rimexolone	1	suspension
Lodeprednol etabonate	0.2–0.5	suspension
	0.5	ointment
Fluorometholone alcohol/acetate	0.1–0.125	suspension
Fluorometholone alcohol	0.1	ointment
Medrysone alcohol	1	solution

Although some animal studies showed corneal penetration differences between prednisolone acetate and sodium phosphate drops, we have not noticed any clinical relevance in everyday practice.

Ophthalmic CS ointments induce lower corneal and anterior chamber drug concentrations than the solutions because the petrolatum vehicle retains the active molecules that are released very slowly. Nevertheless, CS ophthalmic ointments can be an acceptable alternative at night when they remain in the conjunctival fornix in closed eyes with a subsequent prolonged contact time with the ocular surface.

Topical CS administration as a sole therapy usually represents an effective treatment for anterior uveitis but not for intermediate or posterior uveitides except as an adjunct to other therapeutic regimens in case of accompanying anterior segment inflammation such as in panuveitis.

Topical CS route is the treatment of choice for acute (idiopathic or HLA-B27-associated), subacute or chronic (juvenile idiopathic arthritis) anterior uveitis without posterior segment involvement; they can also be indicated for sclerouveitis and some keratouveitis combined with an adequate anti-infectious treatment if there is any doubt on the origin of the corneal involvement.

As we are going to discuss later, in the matter of intraocular inflammation, one must always initiate an intensive treatment from the beginning of the disease. It is recommended for the patient to occlude the lacrimal ducts with the thumb and the forefinger during the 30 s following the instillation of the CS drop in the lower conjunctival fornix in order to avoid systemic absorption particularly in high-frequency application regimen.

In a typical presentation of unilateral idiopathic acute anterior uveitis, the treatment schedule can be as follows (depending on the severity of the intraocular inflammation):

- mydriatics/cycloplegics.
- analgesics, rest.
- topical CS drops (well shaken bottle of 1% prednisolone acetate for example): one drop every 10 min for 1–2 h, then one drop every hour for 1–2 days, then decrease progressively the dosage frequency from one drop 8 times/day to 3 times/day at various time intervals depending upon the clinical response which is unique to each patient. Some patients need to be treated with 1 or 2 drops/day during several weeks or even months. However, one should avoid prolonging such topical treatment more than 3 months; an alternative treatment must be then proposed because of increased risks of adverse effects (glaucoma, cataract). The tapering of topical CS administration can be assisted by repeated Laser Flare Photometry measurements. Progressive tapering can be done initially by decreasing the drops instillation frequency and afterwards by using less and less potent molecules switching from prednisolone acetate to rimexolone and then to lodeprednol.
- during the acute phase, one can concomitantly prescribe a corticosteroids ophthalmic ointment (0.05% dexamethasone sodium phosphate ointment) 3 times/day or only during the night-time.
- If there is no or poor clinical improvement after a relatively short period of topical treatment (2–3 days), one should consider adding a regional and possibly a systemic CS therapy even if the ocular inflammation remains unilateral.

Despite a frequent dosing schedule, the dexamethasone concentration in the aqueous humor is far lower than after a subconjunctival injection with dexamethasone sodium phosphate.

Table 4. Corticosteroids preparations for regional injections (subconjunctival/tenon or transseptal injections)

Drug	Relative Anti-inflammatory Potency	Half-life (hours)	Approximate biologic duration of action	solubility	Dose
Short-acting					
Hydrocortisone	1.0	8–12	1 day	high	50–125 mg
Methylprednisolone sodium succinate	5.0	8–12	1–2 days	high	50–125 mg
Intermediate-acting					
Triamcinolone diacetate	5.0	18–36	2–4 months	intermediate	40 mg
Triamcinolone acetonide	5.0	18–36	2–4 months	intermediate	40 mg
Methylprednisolone acetate	5.0	18–36	2–4 months	intermediate	40–80 mg
Long-acting					
Dexamethasone acetate	25	36–54	7–10 days	low	4–8 mg
Betamethasone acetate/phosphate	25	36–54	7–10 days	low	1–3 mg

Topical CS administration is inefficient for posterior segment inflammatory disorders. The penetration of topical dexamethasone into the vitreous after repeated drop instillations is negligible compared with other administration routes (subconjunctival injection, peribulbar injection or oral administration).

Iontophoresis Technology

It is an active noninvasive method of drug delivery achieving higher drug level inside the eye. A low electric current creates an electrical field promoting the movement of charged substances (drug molecules such as dexamethasone phosphate) across biological membranes (cornea, conjunctiva, episclera). It is currently under investigation for noninfectious anterior uveitis and anterior scleritis.

Regional Preparations and Administration Routes

The most common preparations for periocular injections are listed in table 4.

Periocular steroid injections represent an effective mode of treating uveitis, mostly without inducing steroid systemic side effects. They are particularly indicated in unilateral diseases, in the absence of extraocular inflammatory manifestations, in case of insufficient response to topical CS for the treatment of anterior uveitis.

The advantages of periocular steroids are (1) a high local concentration; (2) a longer duration of action – compared with the topical route – determined by the solubility of the steroid and the location of the injection, and (3) their effectiveness against inflammatory disorders of the posterior segment. The duration and severity of IOP rise is inversely related to the solubility of the injected steroid. Triamcinolone acetonide is a very high-risk agent as it is the least soluble and a long-acting repository steroid. Repeated periocular injections may increase the risk of developing glaucoma.

Periocular injections consist in placing the CS preparation periocularly after topical anesthesia (proparacaine 0.5%, oxybuprocaine 0.4%, tetracaine 0.5–1.0%). Besides repeated topical instillations of anesthetic drops, it is often useful to add in the syringe a local anesthetic (0.1 ml of lidocaine 1%) to the CS preparation. Note that the terms 'peribulbar, periocular or parabulbar injections' are often misused to signify posterior sub-Tenon injections.

The different techniques of periocular injections comprise subconjunctival, peribulbar and retrobulbar injections. They have theoretically different goals:

The subconjunctival and anterior sub-Tenon injections (both are commonly improperly referred to as 'subconjunctival injections') are supposedly aimed to treat anterior segment inflammation and are at higher risk of raised IOP than more posterior injections. In fact, a subconjunctival injection of 2.5 mg of dexamethasone results in a vitreous dexamethasone peak concentration 3 times higher than after a peribulbar injection of 5 mg of dexamethasone and 12 times higher than after an oral dose of 7.5 mg of dexamethasone. The dexamethasone concentration is 11.8 times higher in the aqueous humor than in the vitreous. Thus, a subconjunctival injection is the most effective method for delivering dexamethasone into both the anterior and posterior segments of the eye. Systemic drug absorption following a subconjunctival injection is very high and is similar to the one observed after peribulbar injection.

The posterior sub-Tenon, transseptal (both of them are often commonly referred as 'peri- or parabulbar injections') and retrobulbar injections are thought to be more effective for posterior segment inflammation particularly for macular edema. All three have the same potential to place the drug in the intra- and extraconal spaces. Computed tomography studies have demonstrated the existence of multiple communications between these two compartments, allowing the injected drug to diffuse from one to the other. It is therefore pointless and more dangerous to perform a retrobulbar injection instead of a sub-Tenon injection also known as parabulbar injection.

Generally speaking, the posterior sub-Tenon injection (commonly referred as a 'sub-Tenon injection' as opposed to a 'subconjunctival injection') is performed with a 25- or 27-g, 5/8″ (16-mm) long needle with the bevel towards the globe in the superotemporal quadrant with a side-to-side circumferential motion of the needle in order to verify not entering the sclera while the patient is looking down and nasally; the parabulbar injection usually refers to the deposition of the drug preparation posteriorly, in contact with the sclera, with a gently curved blunt cannula through a small conjunctival/Tenon capsule incision 3–5 mm posterior to the corneoscleral limbus.

Another peribulbar injection technique is called the transseptal injection; it is done through the lower lid at the lateral third of the orbital margin; this technique is comparable to the orbital floor injection.

Summary
Subconjunctival dexamethasone injections (2.5 mg dexamethasone) induce 3 times higher vitreous drug concentrations than peribulbar injections (5.0 mg dexamethasone) [5].

Subconjunctival dexamethasone injections (2.5 mg dexamethasone) induce 12 times higher vitreous drug concentrations than oral administration (7.5 mg dexamethasone).

After a subconjunctival injection, the dexamethasone concentration is 11.8 times higher in the aqueous humor than in the vitreous

Periocular injections (either subconjunctival or peribulbar) are not just a local treatment but can result in significant serum levels comparable to those achieved by a single high oral dose.

The choice of the drug to be injected is dictated by the presentation of the uveitis and the risk factors taking into account the anti-inflammatory potency and the duration of action of the CS preparation. A short-acting CS preparation can be injected once a day for 1–5 days because it disappears in less than 24 h. A long-acting CS preparation can be injected several times over a 1- to 3-month interval; it shows a clinical effect in 2–3 days.

Technique, Indications and Contraindications of Intravitreal Corticosteroids

The technique, indications and contraindications of intravitreal CS injections are described in the chapter by Modorati and Miserocchi [pp. 110–121].

Systemic Preparations

Commonly used preparations for systemic CS therapy are presented in order of increasing anti-inflammatory activity in table 5.

Adjunctive therapy
Adjunctive therapy can prevent some adverse effects particularly during prolonged CS treatments. We tend to give it in all patients on CS treatment whatever the duration or the dosage is. It comprises oral potassium and calcium supplementation, oral vitamin D_3,

Table 5. Systemic CS preparations

Drug	Sodium retention effect	Oral	i.m. or i.v.
Hydrocortisone	1.0	5- to 20-mg tablet 2 mg/ml suspension	25 and 50 mg/ml suspension 100- to 500-mg powder i.m./i.v.
Prednisone	0.8	1-, 5-, 20-, 50-mg tablet 5 mg/ml solution	– –
Prednisolone	0.8	5-, 20-mg tablet, dispersible 15 mg/ml syrup 1 mg/ml, solution	25–100 mg/ml suspension, acetate, i.m. 20 mg/ml solution, sodium phosphate, i.m./i.v.
Methylprednisolone	minimal	2- to 32-mg tablet	40- to 1,000-mg powder, sodium succinate, i.m./i.v. 20–80 mg/ml suspension, acetate, i.m.
Triamcinolone	none	1- to 8-mg tablet, diacetate 4-mg/5-ml syrup, diacetate	10 and 40 mg/ml suspension, acetonide, i.m. 40 mg/ml suspension, diacetate, i.m.
Dexamethasone	minimal	0.25- to 6-mg tablet, sodium 0.5-mg/5-ml solution	4–24 mg/ml solution, sodium phosphate, i.v. 8 mg/ml suspension, acetate, i.m.
Betamethasone	negligible	0.6-mg tablet 0.6-mg/5-ml syrup	3 mg/ml solution, sodium phosphate, i.v. 3 and 6 mg/ml, acetate and sodium phosphate, suspension, i.m.

proton pump inhibitors (omeprazole, pantoprazole) or histamine H_2-receptor antagonist (ranitidine, cimetidine), antiacids, gastric mucosal coating. One must be aware that bisphosphonates can cause uveitis or episcleritis/scleritis in 0.05–0.08% of the patients.

Systemic CS administration

Systemic CS administration can be considered in noninfectious sight-threatening uveitis, particularly when the disease is bilateral and resistant to local therapy.

Induction Therapy. The induction treatment must be aggressive with high doses. The CS administration can be done either by oral or by intravenous route depending on the severity of the inflammation.

In acute sight-threatening inflammation, intravenous pulse CS are usually administered at a dose of 1 g of methylprednisolone per day for 3 consecutive days followed by 0.5–1 mg/kg/day oral prednisone depending upon the severity and the vision threat.

In severe subacute or chronic uveitis, one can treat readily the patient with 1.0–1.2 mg/kg/day of oral prednisone without any previous intravenous pulse CS therapy.

The calculation of the dose according to the weight of the patient is not based on scientific randomized studies. It represents a mean to avoid excessive or insufficient dosage in patients of various weight and size. It also facilitates the adjustment of the treatment along the course of the disease. Thus, one should avoid administering the same average dose of 40 mg/day of oral prednisone to every patient whatever their weight and size are.

Discontinuation and Tapering of Therapy. When the maximum improvement of the inflammation is obtained, one can start to decrease the doses progressively. Sometimes, the intolerance to CS requires discontinuing the treatment. The more the period of CS treatment has been prolonged, the slower the tapering should be. If the patient was treated for only brief periods (less than one month), the treatment may be discontinued rapidly within 1–2 weeks. For certain acute exacerbations of chronic uveitis, glucocorticoids may be administered for a short-term (e.g. for 10–30 days). Administer an initial high dose during the first days of therapy, and then withdraw therapy by tapering the dose over several days.

In contrast, if the CS treatment was administered for a prolonged period of time (more than 1–3 months), one should be very cautious and decrease slowly the doses until complete discontinuation of the CS. This approach will avoid a steroid withdrawal syndrome (of lethargy, fever, myalgia) and a recurrence of the intraocular inflammation with a rebound effect. Many methods of slow withdrawal or 'tapering' have been described.

In one suggested regimen, one can decrease by 2–4 mg prednisone equivalent every 3–7 days until the physiologic dose (4–5 mg of prednisone equivalent) is reached.

Other recommendations state that decrements usually should not exceed 2 mg every 1–2 weeks. Generally, the high initial doses of 1 mg/kg/day of prednisone are decreased relatively rapidly by 5–10 mg/day every 10 days until reaching the dose of 20 mg/day of prednisone. Starting from the dose of 20 mg/day of prednisone, we decrease only by 10% the dose of CS at various time intervals (1, 2 weeks or 1 month or more) until the dose of 10 mg/day of prednisone is reached. Thereafter, we taper the dose by only 1 mg per day every 10–30 days depending on the monitoring of the uveitis. In our institution, we tend to take into account the laser flare photometry for the monitoring of anterior uveitis. For posterior uveitis, we consider primarily the visual function (visual acuity, visual fields), the optical coherence tomography (OCT) and the fundus angiogram results. Indeed, OCT is very informative for the macula area but cannot explore the possible resurgence of chorioretinal inflammation at the periphery during the tapering period.

When a physiologic dosage has been reached, a single oral morning dose of 20 mg of hydrocortisone can be substituted for whatever CS the patient has been receiving. It is recommended to previously check the plasma cortisol levels (at 8.00 a.m. and at 4.00 p.m.), although they are not constantly a reliable indicator of the hypothalamic-pituitary-adrenal axis function. After 2–4 weeks, you may decrease hydrocortisone dosage by 2.5 mg every week until a single morning dosage of 10 mg daily is reached.

In fact, the rate of tapering is dependent upon the disease activity. As there is no validated 'disease activity scoring' system, one should monitor very closely the patient and rely on a set of criteria based on clinical examination and ancillary tests (see further on). The importance of each criterion varies according to the type and severity of the uveitis.

Corticosteroid Dependence. If the intraocular inflammation recurs during the progressively slow tapering of the CS treatment before the complete discontinuation of the CS treatment, particularly if the patient has experienced the same event in the past, one must consider the uveitis as CS dependent. If the threshold needed for controlling the uveitis is above 10 mg/day of prednisone, a CS-sparing agent must be proposed in order to avoid the toxicity of a prolonged CS therapy. If the threshold is below 9–10 mg/day of prednisone, one can consider administering sustained low-dose CS for a prolonged period of time if the treatment is indispensable to maintain a good visual function and to control the intraocular inflammation. This approach must be reevaluated every 6 months with a novel attempt to lower the doses. One can maintain tolerable very low dose CS therapy for several years only if the patient needs less than 7 mg/day of CS. If the uveitis necessitates more than 7 mg/day of prednisone after one year of treatment, one should definitely add a CS-sparing agent.

It must be remembered that one should not wait too long before proposing a combined therapy with a CS-sparing agent. This should be done before the development of CS-induced side effects. Different types of immunomodulatory drugs can be administered in combination with CS. Their choice will depend on the association with extraocular manifestations, the type, the course and the severity of the uveitis.

Corticosteroid Resistance. The uveitis can be 'CS resistant'. High doses of CS cannot control the intraocular inflammation either during the induction treatment or during the tapering of the CS doses. If the inflammation does not respond to the initial intense CS doses (1–1.2 mg/kg/day of prednisone or pulse i.v. methylprednisolone) or to less than 0.5 mg/kg/day during the tapering phase, the uveitis is considered as resistant to CS therapy. A novel workup must be performed, and may be repeated several times in order to exclude an infection or a masquerade syndrome. If a primary intraocular lymphoma is suspected, the CS treatment must be discontinued several weeks before ocular fluid analysis (IL-10 levels in the aqueous humor and in the vitreous, identification of malignant lymphoma cells in the vitreous, gene rearrangement analysis). The exclusion of an infection or a masquerade syndrome is mandatory before starting any immunomodulating treatment.

Indeed, one can also note that some CS-resistant noninfectious uveitis may be responsive to immunomodulatory therapy alone. The absence of response to CS treatment does not preclude the response to immunomodulation. This can justify why, in certain disease entities, the immunomodulatory therapy must be started very early during the course of the uveitis. It is the case in severe noninfectious uveitis associated with extraocular manifestation such as Behçet's disease, or in severe isolated intractable noninfectious uveitis (without systemic inflammatory manifestations) such as birdshot chorioretinopathy.

Alternate-Day Therapy. Alternate-day therapy in which a single dose is administered every other morning is the dosage regimen of choice for long-term oral CS treatment of most conditions. This regimen provides relief of symptoms while minimizing adrenal suppression, protein catabolism, and other adverse effects such as growth retardation. Although an alternate-day dosage regimen is generally insufficient to control long-standing noninfectious uveitis, it can be tempted and proposed in childhood uveitis in order to minimize the incidence of adverse effects, particularly growth retardation. Most authorities consider only a 'short-acting' glucocorticoid that suppresses the hypothalamic-pituitary-adrenal axis less than 1.5 days after a single oral dose (e.g. prednisone, prednisolone, methylprednisolone) to be suitable.

Practical Therapeutic Utilization

General Considerations

CS-intensive induction treatment permits to overcome a difficult threatening phase during the course of the disease. A prolonged maintenance treatment with lower doses is often needed.

As for significant intraocular inflammation, one must always initiate an intensive treatment from the onset of the disease instead of beginning with moderate doses and increase them progressively. Indeed, it is important to control as rapidly as possible the inflammation to avoid irreversible tissue alteration secondary to inflammation and to prevent devastating tissue destruction and scarring. This approach will also shorten the duration of the treatment and decrease the cumulative doses of drug and therefore the risk of developing severe side effects. Moreover, this strategy is clinically valid for infectious (anti-infectious drugs) as well as for noninfectious/autoimmune inflammatory diseases (CS).

Evidently, an aggressive CS therapy cannot be initiated without excluding an infectious etiology. If a doubt still persists on the noninfectious nature of the disease, one should not start CS therapy before administering (several days before beginning the CS treatment) an anti-infectious treatment presumed to cover the suspected infectious etiology. This is the case in self-evolving inflammatory processes following/accompanying an initial infectious trigger in which disease activity can be exacerbated

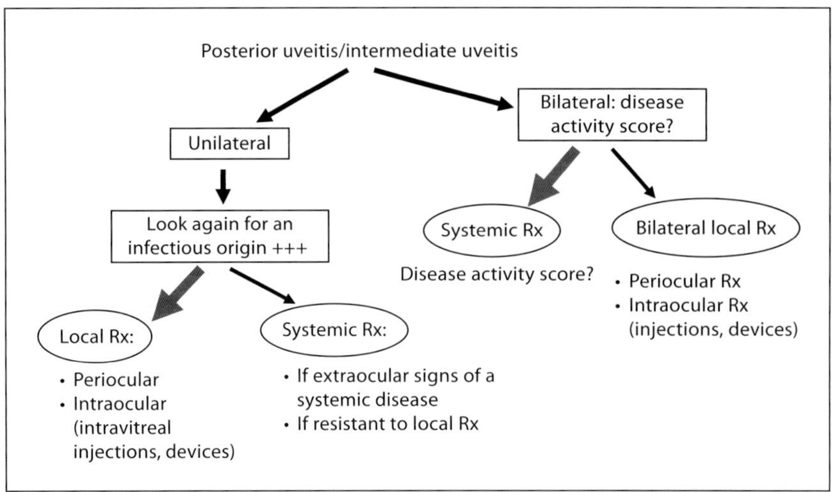

Fig. 2. Corticosteroids: therapeutic strategies (2).

or reactivated by systemic CS alone (toxoplasmosis, Lyme disease, hypersensitivity to *Mycobacterium tuberculosis* proteins for example).

Therapeutic Strategies

Therapeutic strategies are summarized in figures 1–5. The therapeutic decision depends upon the type, the uni-/bilaterality and the course of the uveitis.

It is difficult to standardize the management of uveitis in general because of the lack of a validated 'disease activity score' particularly for posterior uveitis. Most of the therapeutic regimens are given according to the physician's clinical judgment. There is no standard treatment because of the heterogeneity of clinical responses for the 'same' apparent disease. However, it is still important to base the therapeutic adjustment on objective criteria. We used a combination of factors: clinical examination, laser flare photometry, OCT, fundus angiograms (fluorescein and indocyanine green), visual fields. Obviously, the visual acuity must not be the only criteria.

In most of the cases, a unilateral anterior uveitis can be treated locally by drops and subconjunctival CS injections which induce higher aqueous humor CS concentrations than peribulbar/parabulbar CS injections. Although it can induce significant CS serum levels on a short-term, the local treatment causes much less side effects than a systemic CS administration. When the uveitis is unilateral, it is very important to exclude an infectious etiology before any CS application (fig. 1, 2). The physician may decide to give a systemic treatment if she/he considers that the intraocular inflammation is not efficiently controlled by the local treatment and in the case of accompanying extraocular manifestations of a systemic disease. In severe bilateral anterior

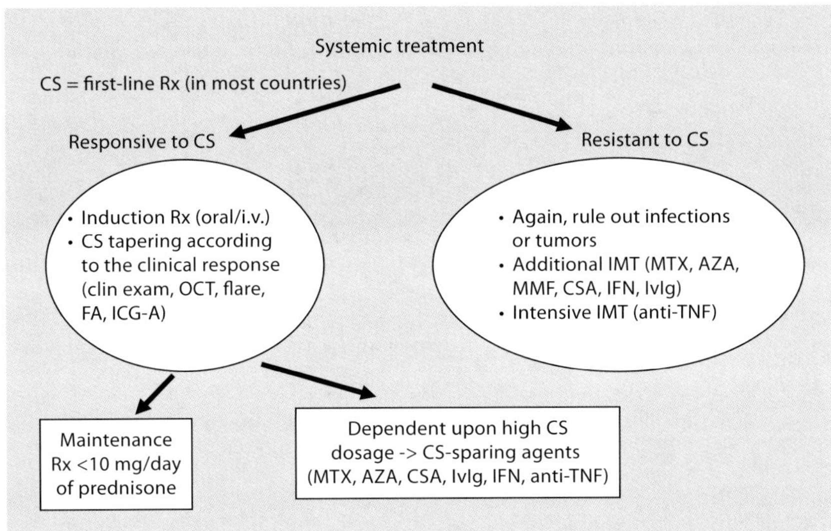

Fig. 3. Corticosteroids: therapeutic strategies (3). FA = Fluorescein angiography; ICG-A = indocyanine green angiography; IMT = immunomodulatory treatment; MTX = methotrexate; AZA = azathioprine; MMF = mycophenolate mofetil; CSA = cyclosporine; IFN = interferon; Ivlg = intravenous immunoglobulins.

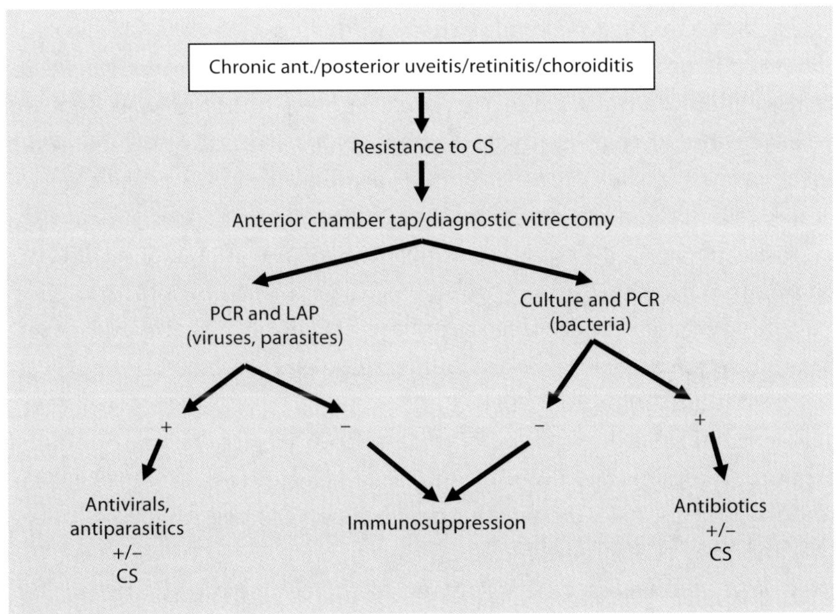

Fig. 4. Corticosteroids: therapeutic strategies (4). LAP = Local Antibody Production.

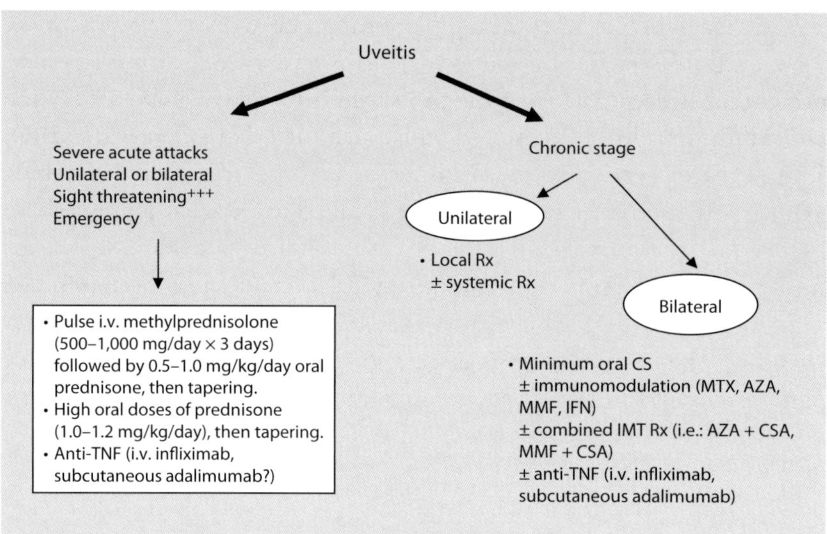

Fig. 5. Corticosteroids: therapeutic strategies (5).

uveitis, a bilateral intensive local treatment is rapidly efficient most of the time, but a combination of local and systemic CS treatment is often used in order to shorten the duration of such a disabling condition.

Unlike bilateral anterior uveitis, one tends to use more often a systemic therapeutic approach for bilateral posterior uveitis rather than a bilateral local treatment (fig. 2). In posterior uveitis, which are more often chronic and long-standing than anterior uveitis (there are exceptions such as in juvenile idiopathic arthritis for example, even though the anterior uveitis can be controlled with topical CS and rarely needs periocular CS injections), it is difficult to repeat bilateral periocular injections for a prolonged period of time. The systemic treatment has also the advantage of modifying the immune and inflammatory response upstream of the eye itself by a direct action on the general immune system. Local treatments are acting only at the end of the chain, although, as already said, a periocular CS injection can induce CS serum levels equivalent to an oral systemic administration.

If the intraocular inflammation is resistant to a proper CS treatment, one must again rule out an underlying infection or a masquerade syndrome before proceeding with immunomodulation (fig. 3, 4). Ocular fluid analysis is very helpful for excluding an infection (local antibody production, PCR, culture).

The therapeutic approach is different according to the course of the disease (fig. 5). During a sight-threatening acute attack, we tend to use the intravenous route (pulse i.v. methylprednisolone or i.v. anti-TNF agents), although there is no evidence that pulse i.v. CS give a better outcome than high-dose oral CS. However, the clinical impression is that the intraocular inflammation seems to subside more rapidly after i.v. pulse than oral CS.

During the chronic stage of a long-standing non-infectious uveitis, the minimum CS treatment must be administered. The goal is to determine the CS threshold needed to control the intraocular inflammation. If the threshold is too high, above 7 mg/day of prednisone, an immunomodulatory therapy must be added. For unilateral uveitis, a repeated local treatment should be favored knowing that the adjunction of a low-dose systemic therapy can sometimes decrease the frequency and the dosing of the local treatment.

New therapeutic approaches [corticosteroid intravitreal devices and implants; see the chapter by de Smet, pp. 122–133] are now available for treating noninfectious uveitis locally, avoiding the severe adverse effects of a systemic treatment. Those novel methods are particularly interesting in unilateral cases without extraocular manifestations.

Adverse Effects of Corticosteroid Therapy

CS associated adverse effects are dependent on both the average dose and the duration of therapy. Even low-dose CS therapy could lead to serious adverse effects [6].

Ocular Side Effects of Corticosteroid Treatment

General Considerations

Ocular side effects following systemic administration include [7]: posterior subcapsular cataract (cataracts 15%, and fractures 12% were among the most serious adverse effects of long-term CS therapy), increased IOP/glaucoma, increased susceptibility to infection, reactivation of viral diseases (i.e. herpes group), impaired corneal wound healing, corneal/scleral thinning, subconjunctival hemorrhage, myopia, proptosis, diplopia, extraocular muscle paresis, ptosis, eyelid edema, visual hallucinations, abnormal electroretinogram/visual evoked potential, optic disc edema, central serous chorioretinopathy, iris/ciliary body microcysts.

The threshold for the increase in IOP was observed at dosages of over 7.5 mg/day of prednisone. A very low threshold was observed for eye cataract (<5 mg/day of prednisone).

Ocular side effects following topical or periocular administration are: cataract, increased IOP/glaucoma (a patient's negative response to topical steroids does not predict the response to periocular steroids), increased susceptibility to infection, impaired corneal/scleral wound healing, corneal/scleral thinning, subconjunctival hemorrhage/hematoma, superficial punctate keratitis, corneal deposits, paresis of accommodation, extraocular muscle paresis, ptosis, strabismus, accidental intraocular injection.

Ocular side effects following intravitreal injections include [for more details, see the chapter by de Smet, pp. 122–133]: pain, impaired visual acuity/floaters, elevated

IOP/glaucoma is frequent (>50%), retinal/vitreous hemorrhage, retinal tear/detachment, endophthalmitis, elevated risk of infectious retinitis.

Whatever the route of CS administration is, the two main frequent issues are the rise in IOP and the development of cataract.

Intraocular Pressure Elevation

CS have been shown to cause an elevation in IOP through all modes of administration. The rise in IOP usually occurs over a period of 4–7 weeks if used topically and months or years if used systemically. There have been some reports of an elevation of IOP within hours of initiating intensive topical steroid use.

Some modes of administration can be discontinued easily, thereby reducing or reversing any untoward effects on IOP. Other modes of administration, however, such as sub-Tenon's, or intravitreal injections, are not as easily reversed if problems arise.

'Steroid responder' patients represent 5–6% of the normal population; they develop a marked increase of IOP of more than 16 mm Hg after 4–6 weeks of topical steroid administration, while 30% of the population have a rise of 6–15 mm Hg. Monitoring IOP in all patients receiving steroids is necessary. Once the steroids have been stopped, the IOP almost always returns to baseline within 4 weeks [8–10].

A sub-Tenon injection of a CS preparation with depot effect induces much more frequently an elevation of the IOP than when using a non-depot CS preparation. A rise in IOP ≥5 mm Hg was found in 46% of the eyes, and an IOP >21 mm Hg was found in 30% of the eyes after a single injection of triamcinolone. The IOP increased within 3 months in 81% of the eyes and after 4 months in 19% of the eyes. The IOP began to increase significantly from 2 weeks up to 5 months and returned to the baseline IOP in 10 months. The incidence of IOP elevation ≥5 mm Hg or an IOP of >21 mm Hg after multiple sub-Tenon injections of triamcinolone was significantly higher than after a single injection (62 and 47%, respectively) [11]. IOP elevation occurs in 21% of the patients after sub-Tenon triamcinolone injections for noninfectious uveitis with a clinical improvement in 52% of the cases [12].

CS-induced glaucoma is more frequent in some patients: children, elderly, patients with higher baseline IOP, patient or family history of primary open angle glaucoma, high myopia, diabetes mellitus, connective tissue disease, traumatic angle recession glaucoma, Cushing's syndrome, high doses of subtenon CS injection [13, 14].

Management consists of discontinuation of steroids, medical therapy and/or surgical intervention. Recent studies showed that prostaglandin analogs may be used in uveitic glaucoma patients [15].

IOP elevation is related to steroid type, potency, dose, duration and route of administration. The steroid types inducing glaucoma are in ascending order: medrysone, hydrocortisone, fluorometholone, rimexolone, prednisolone/prednisone, dexamethasone/betamethasone. The routes of administration inducing glaucoma are in ascending order: systemic, topical, subtenon (depot preparation), subconjunctival (depot preparation), intravitreal (depot preparation).

Corticosteroid-Induced Cataract Formation

The incidence of posterior subcapsular cataract is related to the duration and the dose of CS therapy. If the patient was treated less than one year, there was no CS-induced cataract whatever the dose of CS treatment was (even for doses as high as 60 mg/day of prednisone). During CS treatment lasting between 1 and 4 years, doses below 10 mg/day of prednisone did not induce cataract formation. The incidence of cataract formation increased to 11% for doses between 10 and 15 mg/day of prednisone and to 78% for doses above 16 mg/day of prednisone. If low-dose CS treatment ≥3 mg/day is prolonged more than 4 years, the incidence of cataract is 83% [16].

The incidence of cataract formation after one subtenon triamcinolone injection varies from 2.1 to 18% within 12 months following the injection depending on different series [17, 18].

In children with juvenile idiopathic arthritis-related uveitis, the chronic use of topical CS dosed at ≤3 drops daily was associated with an 87% lower risk of cataract formation compared with eyes treated with >3 drops daily independently of uveitis activity [19].

Nonocular Side Effects of Corticosteroid Treatment

The nonocular adverse effects of CS therapy are as outlined below.

Fluid and electrolyte disturbances: Sodium retention, fluid retention, congestive heart failure in susceptible patients, potassium loss, hypokalemic alkalosis, hyperosmolar coma, hypertension. We recommend a salt-free diet above 10 mg/day of oral prednisone.

Musculoskeletal: Muscle weakness, steroid myopathy, loss of muscle mass, osteoporosis, vertebral compression fractures, aseptic necrosis of femoral and humeral heads, pathologic fracture of long bones, tendon rupture. Risk of osteoporosis on long-term CS is as follows: prednisone 1–5 mg: relative risk 1.9×; prednisone 5–10 mg: relative risk 4.5×; prednisone >10 mg: relative risk 32×.

Recommended lifestyle measures from day 1 of CS treatment: smoking cessation, weight-bearing and strength-building exercises, calcium intake of 1,000–1,500 mg per day, vitamin D 800–1,000 IU/day.

Bisphosphonates are effective and recommended, but one must be aware that they can induce anterior uveitis and episcleritis/scleritis in rare cases.

Gastrointestinal: Peptic ulcer with possible subsequent perforation and hemorrhage of small and large bowel; pancreatitis; abdominal distention; ulcerative esophagitis; nausea; increased appetite.

Dermatologic: Impaired wound healing, thin fragile skin; petechiae and ecchymoses; facial erythema; increased sweating; may suppress reactions to skin tests.

Neurological: Convulsions; increased intracranial pressure with papilledema (pseudotumor cerebri) usually after treatment; vertigo; headaches; insomnia.

Psychiatric effects: Patients and/or carers should be warned that potentially severe psychiatric reactions may occur. Symptoms typically emerge within a few days or weeks of starting treatment. Most reactions recover after either dose reduction or withdrawal, although specific treatment may be necessary. Patients and/or carers should be encouraged to seek medical advice if worrying psychological symptoms develop, especially if depressed mood or suicidal ideation is suspected. Particular care is required when considering the use of CS in patients with existing or previous history of severe affective disorders. Psychic derangements range from euphoria, insomnia, mood swings, hyperexcitability, personality changes and severe depression to frank psychotic manifestations.

Endocrine: Menstrual irregularities; development of cushingoid state; suppression of growth in children; secondary adrenocortical and pituitary unresponsiveness, particularly in times of stress, as in trauma, surgery, or illness; decreased carbohydrate tolerance; hirsutism; manifestations of latent diabetes mellitus; increased requirements for insulin or oral hypoglycemic agents in diabetics. We recommend a diet without quick-burning sugars.

Metabolic: Negative nitrogen balance due to protein catabolism; centripetal obesity.

Immunologic: Impaired inflammatory response.

Other: Weight gain; hypertension; thromboembolism.

The following additional adverse reactions are related to parenteral and intralesional corticosteroid therapy: rare instances of blindness associated with intralesional therapy around the face and head; hyperpigmentation or hypopigmentation; subcutaneous and cutaneous atrophy; sterile abscess; anaphylactoid reactions have been rarely reported.

High-Risk Group of Patients

Pregnancy

CS have been shown to be teratogenic in many species when given in doses equivalent to the human dose. Animal studies in which CS have been given to pregnant mice, rats, and rabbits have yielded an increased incidence of cleft palate in the offspring. There are no adequate and well-controlled studies in pregnant women. CS should be used during pregnancy only if the potential benefit justifies the potential risk to the fetus. Infants born to mothers who have received CS during pregnancy should be carefully observed for signs of hypoadrenalism. The final decision depends on the benefit/risk ratio and should be discussed with the patient's gynecologist.

Use in Lactation
CS appear in breast milk and could suppress growth, interfere with endogenous CS production or cause other unwanted effects in breastfed infants. Women taking CS should be advised not to breastfeed.

Use in Children
CS cause growth retardation in infancy, childhood and adolescence, which may be irreversible and therefore long-term administration of pharmacological doses should be avoided. If prolonged therapy is necessary, treatment should be limited to the minimum suppression of the hypothalamo-pituitary adrenal axis and growth retardation, the growth and development of infants and children should be closely monitored. Treatment should be administered when possible as a single dose on alternate days. Children are at special risk from raised intracranial pressure.

Use in the Elderly
Long-term use in the elderly should be planned bearing in mind the more serious consequences of the common side effects of CS in old age, especially osteoporosis, diabetes, hypertension, hypokalemia, susceptibility to infection and thinning of the skin. Close medical supervision is required to avoid life-threatening reactions.

Conclusion

CS are considered to be the mainstay of therapy in noninfectious uveitis. Their indications depend upon numerous factors, among them the type (involving or not the posterior segment), the severity, the uni-/bilaterality, the chronicity of the intraocular inflammation. CS should not be used at high doses as a sole treatment in the long-term because of severe adverse effects. The goal is to find, for each individual patient, the minimum CS dose necessary for controlling the intraocular inflammation. If the threshold of CS dependence is too high, an infectious origin has to be considered and must be excluded again by a novel complete workup. The exclusion of an infection and of a masquerade syndrome is mandatory before starting an immunomodulating treatment for sparing the CS dosage. Although CS administration by various routes is the first line of therapy for noninfectious uveitis, it cannot remain the sole prolonged treatment in long-standing diseases in the majority of the cases.

Combining immunomodulating agents with low-dose CS is the preferred regimen for controlling intraocular inflammation with a minimum of side effects when long-term therapy is needed.

References

1 Stewart PM: The adrenal cortex. In: Kronenberg HM, Melmed S, Polonsky KS, Larsen RP (eds). Williams Textbook of Endocrinology, 11th ed. Philadelphia, PA, Saunders; 2008, Chapter 14.

2 Vitale AT, Foster CS: Corticosteroids. In Foster CS, Vitale AT, editors: Diagnosis and Treatment of Uveitis, Philadelphia, WB Saunders; 2002. Chapter 9, pp 142–157.

3 Nussenblatt RB, Whitcup SM: Philosophy, goals, and approaches to medical therapy. In Nussenblatt RB, Whitcup SM: Uveitis, Fundamentals and Clinical Practice, Mosby-Elsevier; 2010. Chapter 7, pp 77–84.

4 Cunningham ET Jr, Wender JD: Practical approach to the use of corticosteroids in patients with uveitis. Can J Ophthalmol 2010;45:352–358.

5 Weijtens O, Feron EJ, Schoemaker RC, Cohen AF, Lentjes EG, Romijn FP, van Meurs JC: High concentration of dexamethasone in aqueous and vitreous after subconjunctival injection. Am J Ophthalmol 1999;128:192–197.

6 Curtis JR, Westfall AO, Allison J, Bijlsma JW, Freeman A, George V, Kovac SH, Spettell CM, Saag KG: Population-based assessment of adverse events associated with long-term glucocorticoid use. Arthritis Rheum 2006;55:420–426.

7 Fraunfelder FT, Fraunfelder FW, Chambers WA: Hormones and agents affecting hormonal mechanisms. In Fraunfelder FT, Fraunfelder FW, Chambers WA (eds): Clinical Ocular Toxicology, Saunders Elsevier; 2008. Chapter 7, pp 169–173.

8 Armaly MF: Statistical attributes of the steroid hypertensive response in the clinically normal eye. Invest Ophthalmol Vis Sci 1965;4:187–197.

9 Becker B: Intraocular pressure response to topical corticosteroids. Invest Ophthalmol Vis Sci 1965;4:198–205.

10 Becker B, Mills DW: Corticosteroids and intraocular pressure. Arch Ophthalmol 1963;70:500–507.

11 Kawamura R, Inoue M, Shinoda H, Shinoda K, Itoh Y, Ishida S, Tsubota K: Incidence of increased intraocular pressure after subtenon injection of triamcinolone acetonide. J Ocul Pharmacol Ther 2011;27:299–304.

12 Bui Quoc E, Bodaghi B, Adam R, Burtin T, Cassoux N, Dreifuss S, Fardeau C, LeHoang P: Intraocular pressure elevation after subtenon injection of triamcinolone acetonide during uveitis (in French). J Fr Ophtalmol 2002;25:1048–1056.

13 Jones III R, Rhee DJ: Corticosteroid-induced ocular hypertension and glaucoma: a brief review and update of the literature; Curr Opin Ophthalmol 2006;17:163–167.

14 Tripathi RC, Parapuram SK, Tripathi BJ, Zhong Y, Chalam KV: Corticosteroids and glaucoma risk. Drugs Aging 1999;15:439–450.

15 Sallam A, Sheth HG, Habot-Wilner Z, Lightman S: Outcome of raised intraocular pressure in uveitic eyes with and without a corticosteroid-induced hypertensive response. Am J Ophthalmol 2009;148: 207e1–213e1.

16 Urban RC Jr, Cotlier E: Corticosteroid-induced cataracts. Surv Ophthalmol 1986;31:102–110.

17 Yoshimura M, Hirano Y, Nozaki M, Yoshida M, Ogura Y: Incidence of posterior subcapsular cataract progression after triamcinolone acetonide administration (in Japanese). Nihon Ganka Gakkai Zasshi 2008;112:786–789.

18 Byun YS, Park YH: Complications and safety profile of posterior subtenon injection of triamcinolone acetonide. J Ocul Pharmacol Ther 2009;25:159–162.

19 Thorne JE, Woreta FA, Dunn JP, Jabs DA: Risk of cataract development among children with juvenile idiopathic arthritis-related uveitis treated with topical corticosteroids. Ophthalmology 2010;117: 1436–1441.

Phuc LeHoang
Department of Ophthalmology
University of Paris VI
Pitié-Salpêtrière Hospital
83 Boulevard de L'Hôpital
FR–75013 Paris (France)
E-Mail phuc.lehoang@psl.ap-hop-paris.fr

Miserocchi E, Modorati G, Foster CS (eds): New Treatments in Noninfectious Uveitis.
Dev Ophthalmol. Basel, Karger, 2012, vol 51, pp 29–46

Corticosteroid-Sparing Agents: Conventional Systemic Immunosuppressants

Jonathan Kruh · C. Stephen Foster

Massachusetts Eye Research and Surgery Institution, Ocular Immunology and Uveitis Foundation, Cambridge, Mass., USA

Abstract

The introduction of corticosteroids in the mid-20th century to control inflammatory eye disease revolutionized treatment practices. As long-term use of corticosteroids became the backbone of immunosuppressive therapy, it soon became evident that it was associated with significant morbidity to the patient. For this reason, other immunosuppressant agents were sought. Thereafter, the first generation of immunosuppressive agents were born. The main action of all such agents involves the inhibition of lymphoid proliferation. The agents can be further subdivided into the following categories based on their specific mechanism of action: alkylating (cyclophosphamide and chlorambucil), antimetabolite (methotrexate, mycophenolate mofetil and azathioprine), and antibiotic/calcineurin inhibitor (cyclosporine, tacrolimus and sirolimus). These immunomodulating agents serve as the foundation to modern corticosteroid-sparing immunosuppressive therapy. Many times, these agents are now even indicated as first-line therapy for the treatment of systemic inflammatory diseases with destructive ocular sequela, e.g. Behçet's disease and granulomatosis with polyangiitis (Wegener's). Choosing the most appropriate immunomodulatory agent to initiate therapy can often be difficult; a multifactorial approach in the decision-making process is essential. Special attention must be given to the patient's medical history, type and severity of inflammatory disease, social history, compliance, age, and sex. Oftentimes, it takes a joint effort between the ophthalmologist and multiple sub-specialists (rheumatology, oncology, and hematology) to administer and monitor these therapies. Even though each of these systemic immunosuppressive agents has its own array of potential side effects, with careful monitoring and titration of dosages, such potential side effects can be minimized or avoided altogether. Ultimately, these patients are afforded a much more favorable long-term outcome, free of the devastating effects of chronic corticosteroid use.

Indications & Dosage

For an overview of the drugs to be discussed in this chapter, see Tables 1 and 2.

Table 1. Major indications for the use of conventional immunosuppressive drugs

Drug	Indications
Cyclophosphamide	granulomatosis with polyangiitis (Wegener's), polyarteritis nodosa, necrotizing scleritis, scleritis associated with rheumatoid arthritis or polychondritis, Mooren's ulcer, cicatricial pemphigoid, sympathetic ophthalmia, ABD
Chlorambucil	ABD, sympathetic ophthalmia, JIA associated with iridocyclitis
Methotrexate	sympathetic ophthalmia, scleritis, JIA associated with iridocyclitis
Azathioprine	ABD, granulomatosis with polyangiitis (Wegener's), systemic lupus erythematosus, scleritis, cicatricial pemphigoid, JIA associated with iridocyclitis
CSA	ABD, birdshot retinochoroidopathy, sarcoidosis, pars planitis, VKH syndrome, sympathetic ophthalmia, idiopathic posterior uveitis, corneal graft rejection

Table 2. Suggested dosing for medications

Medication	Dose	Administration
Cyclophosphamide	1–3 mg/kg/day	oral, intravenous
Chlorambucil	0.1 mg/kg/day	oral
Methotrexate	0.15 mg/kg once weekly	oral, intramuscular
Azathioprine	1–3 mg/kg/day	oral
Cyclosporine	2.5–5 mg/kg/day	oral

Alkylating Agents

Alkylating agents are so named because of their ability to form covalent bonds (alkylation) with neutrophilic substances. Specifically, they function by attaching an alkyl group onto 7-nitrogen guanine [1].

Cyclophosphamide (Cytoxan®, Neosar®)

History and Source

Cyclophosphamide is a member of the nitrogen mustard family of alkylating agents. The first use of nitrogen mustard predates its medicinal applications. This agent was first used for chemical warfare during World War I. At the time, it was found that exposure to nitrogen mustard had profound effects on the bone marrow, causing leukopenia and aplasia of lymphoid tissue [2]. Although, it was not until the 1950s when its application for the treatment of uveitis was first reported by Roda-Perez [3–5].

Pharmacology

Cyclophosphamide is a prodrug converted by the hepatic microsomal cytochrome P-450 mixed function oxidase system into its active metabolites phosphoramide mustard and 4-hydroxycyclophosphamide [6]. Through nucleophillic substitution reactions, these metabolites form covalent cross-linkages with DNA. It is through alkylation with DNA that this agent has its immunosuppressive function. The active form of cyclophosphamide targets the 7-nitrogen atom of guanine, which promotes guanine-thymidine linkages. Ultimately, this leads to miscoding, breaks in single-stranded DNA, and the formation of phosphodiester bonds after repair of those breaks, with subsequent defective cell function [7]. These interactions occur between both DNA and RNA, and are cell-cycle nonspecific [8].

Clinical Pharmacology

In its clinical application, cyclophosphamide has been found to have depressive actions on both B and T cell populations. With acute administration of high doses, B cells are more specifically targeted [9]. However, when treated at lower doses, and more chronically, both B and T cells are equally affected [10, 11]. The effects on the humoral arm of the immune system result in suppression of both primary and secondary antibody responses [9, 12, 13]. Additionally, it is effective in inhibiting cell-mediated immunity [8]. Finally, it aids in the inhibition of monocyte precursors.

Therapeutic Value

Even though there can be the potential for significant toxicity from cyclophosphamide therapy, it still maintains an important role in the treatment of many inflammatory diseases, especially when recalcitrant to other therapies. In particular, cyclophosphamide is the treatment of choice for patients with ocular disease from granulomatosis with polyangiitis (Wegener's) and polyarteritis nodosa. When used as either monotherapy or as adjuvant treatment with corticosteroids, it can be invaluable in improving both patient survival as well as maintaining ocular integrity [14–17]. Bilateral Mooren's ulcer, often nonresponsive to more conventional treatments may have good response to cyclophosphamide therapy. Significant recovery rates and improved outcomes in patients with aggressive bilateral Mooren's ulcer have been reported by Foster, Brown and Mondino [18, 19]. In patients with active ocular cicatricial pemphigoid, cyclophosphamide may also be considered a first-line agent [20]. The evidence for this was supported by Foster in a randomized, double-masked, clinical trial proving the superiority of combination treatment with cyclophosphamide and prednisone versus prednisone alone [20]. The efficacy of cyclophosphamide over corticosteroid monotherapy for the treatment of ocular manifestations of Adamantiades-Behçet's Disease (ABD) has also been reported in the literature [21]. Both cyclophosphamide and chlorambucil were also shown to be superior to cyclosporine in the treatment of ABD [22]. Other ocular inflammatory disorders that are often refractory to treatment with prednisone and other immunosuppressive agents, but successfully treated with cyclophosphamide, include pars planitis and sympathetic ophthalmia [23, 24].

Dosage and Side Effects

Cyclophosphamide may be given orally, intramuscularly, intravenously, intrapleurally, or intraperitoneally. Orally, ~75% is absorbed in the gastrointestinal tract. It reaches peak plasma levels within 1 h of ingestion and can be found distributed throughout the body, including the brain [25]. Cyclophosphamide undergoes conversion to its cytotoxic metabolites in the liver. These active metabolites are 50% bound to plasma albumin. The plasma half-life of cyclophosphamide is 4–6 h. Ultimately, ~10–20% of the native drug is excreted in the urine unchanged [26].

There are numerous side effects that patients may encounter when being treated with cyclophosphamide. The array and severity of side effects that one might experience is usually dose related. The most frequent complaint from patients is gastrointestinal upset. This may manifest as anorexia, nausea, vomiting, or stomatitis [26]. Oftentimes, when this medication is given intravenously, this side effect can be decreased by giving prophylactic ondansetron.

The most common dose-limiting effect from cyclophosphamide is bone marrow depression. Leukocytes are significantly affected, more commonly than platelets. Leukopenia and/or thrombocytopenia has a peak incidence 1–2 weeks after i.v. therapy, and usually resolves within 10 days after the last received dose [1]. Often trimethoprim-sulfamethoxazole is given prophylactically to prevent pneumocystis pneumonia, a complication found in immunosuppressed individuals.

Another serious potential side effect is gonadal dysfunction. Azoospermia and amenorrhea can be found in 60% of individuals after 6 months of treatment [27]. Since this is often irreversible, sperm or ovum banking is suggested for those who wish to have children.

If one is on oral cyclophosphamide therapy, we suggest that it be taken in the morning, and that the patient consume 3–4 l of fluids throughout the day, in order to promote frequent voiding. Active metabolites (acrolein) in the bladder cause irritation of the mucosa which may lead to hemorrhagic cystitis and to malignant transformation of bladder epithelium, leading to bladder cancer. This may occur as early as 24 h after initiation and as late as several weeks after suspension of therapy [1]. Most often, this complication resolves with discontinuation of the drug, high fluid intake, and bed rest. In rare but severe cases, supravesical urinary diversion may be required [28]. On the other hand, i.v. therapy is often the preferred method of administration because it allows for rapid induction, decreased rates of hemorrhagic cystitis, and transient neutropenia, making infections less frequent.

Table 3. Special considerations for cyclophosphamide

Contraindications to treatment • Patients receiving other concurrent immunosuppressive therapy for an independent reason; e.g. previous radiation therapy, tumor cell infiltration of the bone marrow, or previous cytotoxic therapy • Patients with focal chorioretinitis, herpes simplex, herpes zoster, CMV, AIDS retinopathy, toxoplasmosis, tuberculosis, and fungal infections • Those with a severely depressed bone marrow function • Hypersensitivity to the drug • Pregnancy class D • Excreted in breast milk
Drug interactions • The metabolism of cyclophosphamide is affected by drugs that interact with the P-450 mixed-function oxidase system

Other possible side effects range from alopecia, dry eye, increased intraocular pressure, cardiac myopathy, hepatic dysfunction, irreversible pulmonary fibrosis, impaired renal clearance of water with resultant hyponatremia, and anaphylaxis [25, 26, 29] (see table 3).

Systemic Immunosuppressive Therapy for Eye Disease Study
Cyclophosphamide was not found to be significantly associated with an increase in the incidence of mortality (fully adjusted hazard ratio 1.14, 95% CI 0.81–1.60), but was found to be non-significantly associated with an increase in cancer-related mortality (fully adjusted hazard ratio 1.61, 95% CI 0.81–3.22) [see 50, 51]. These results corroborate evidence from other studies which support that there is an association with the development of secondary malignancies, specifically acute myelocytic leukemia, bladder cancer and skin cancer [30–33].

Chlorambucil

History and Source
Chlorambucil was first created in the 1950s, and was primarily used for the treatment of malignant lymphoma [3]. Its role in the ophthalmic world came about in 1970 when Mamo and Azzam [34] first reported its use and efficacy for the treatment of ABD.

Pharmacology
Chlorambucil is a nitrogen mustard derivative. Likewise, its affect as an alkylating agent is similar to that of cyclophosphamide. Its functions are cell-cycle nonspecific,

Table 4. Special considerations for chlorambucil

Contraindications to treatment
• No known drug-to-drug interactions
• Hypersensitivity to drug
• Pregnancy class D
• Unknown excretion into breast milk

as it impedes both DNA replication and RNA transcription [7, 8]. As an unmetabolized prodrug, chlorambucil is both plasma and tissue bound. Like cyclophosphamide, this prodrug is metabolized into its active form in the liver. There, it is converted to its active metabolite, phenylacetic acid. The major route of excretion is through the kidney [26].

Clinical Pharmacology

The immunosuppressive effect of chlorambucil is manifested through B cell suppression. Of the nitrogen mustard-based agents, it is the slowest acting, taking up to 2 weeks to have an effect [35].

Therapeutic Value

Since its first use for ABD by Mamo and Azzam, chlorambucil has shown great efficacy in the treatment of active ABD by many other investigators [34, 36–40]. It also has been shown to allow for long-term remission of this disease [41, 42]. This agent may also have a significant role in the treatment of juvenile idiopathic arthritis (JIA)-associated iridocyclitis, and sympathetic ophthalmia [24, 43–46].

Dosage and Side Effects

Expectedly, chlorambucil has a similar side effect profile to cyclophosphamide. The most prominent of these is bone marrow suppression. Under normal circumstances, myelosuppression is moderate, gradual, and reversible. However, persistent leukopenia, requiring many months for resolution following discontinuation of the drug, has also been reported. This is most notable in patients who had been receiving high doses of this drug [47].

Other notable side effects include gonadal dysfunction, gastrointestinal upset, cystitis, pulmonary fibrosis, hepatitis, rash, and CNS stimulation (i.e. seizures) [1, 48, 49] (see table 4).

Systemic Immunosuppressive Therapy for Eye Disease Study

Chlorambucil was not found to be associated with an increased incidence of mortality (fully adjusted hazard ratio: 1.43, 95% CI 0.72–2.85), but was found to be significantly associated with an increase in cancer-related mortality (fully adjusted hazard ratio: 2.29, 95% CI 0.53–9.83) [50, 51]. These results appear to be in line with other reports, which suggest a correlation between chlorambucil and the incidence of acute myelogenous leukemia [33, 52, 53].

Antimetabolites

Antimetabolites are chemicals that act to inhibit the functionality of a metabolite. Disabling a metabolite prevents the completion of a pathway in an enzymatic/metabolic reaction [54].

Methotrexate

History and Source
Methotrexate made its debut in 1948, first reported for the treatment of acute leukemia in children [55]. Today, in addition to acute lymphocytic leukemia, it is utilized to treat a variety of systemic inflammatory diseases. These include psoriasis, rheumatoid arthritis, JIA, reactive arthritis, polymyositis, and sarcoidosis [8, 56, 57]. The efficacy of methotrexate for the treatment of ocular inflammatory disease was first reported by Wong and Hersh in 1965 [58]. Since that time, it is often regarded as the first line agent when starting a patient with uveitis on immunosuppressive therapy.

Pharmacology
Methotrexate is analogous in structure to folic acid, excluding two areas; the amino group in the 4-carbon position is substituted for a hydroxyl group, and a methyl group is substituted for a hydrogen atom at the n-1 position [8, 59]. It acts as an irreversible, competitive inhibitor of the enzyme dihydrofolate reductase. The disruption of this enzymatic pathway prevents the conversion of dihydrofolate to tetrahydrofolate, an essential cofactor in the synthesis of the purine nucleotides and thymidylate [7]. Additionally, methotrexate offers partial, reversible, competitive inhibition of thymidylate synthetase. Ultimately, DNA synthesis, repair, RNA synthesis, and cell division (S-phase cell cycle specific) are inhibited.

Clinical Pharmacology
Methotrexate targets cells that are actively dividing. Thus, rapidly dividing cell populations are most dramatically affected, e.g. malignant cells, fetal cells, cells of the gastrointestinal tract, urinary bladder, buccal mucosa, and bone marrow.

Methotrexate suppresses both B and T cells. At low doses, it has little effect on cell-mediated immunity, but has been shown to depress acute-phase reactants [60,

61]. Therefore, it is suspected that the action of methotrexate is more likely anti-inflammatory than immunosuppressive [62].

Therapeutic Value

In the early years following the advent of methotrexate use, it was sparsely used in fear of its adverse side effects. Initial case studies by Wong proved it efficacious in treating steroid-resistant uveitis and sympathetic ophthalmia [58, 63, 64]. But it was the fields of rheumatology and dermatology that paved the way for widespread acceptability of this medication. At lower doses and decreased frequencies, it was found that there could be significant benefits to patients with inflammatory disorders with fewer of the serious side effects [65]. Methotrexate is now used to control scleritis associated with collagen vascular diseases, such as reactive arthritis and rheumatoid arthritis, but not disease complicated by relapsing polyangiitis [66]. In particular, it has been found that weekly dosing either orally or intramuscularly may be effective for the treatment of reactive arthritis, ankylosing spondylitis, psoriatic arthritis, and JIA [8, 45]. Although not as effective as monotherapy for retinal vasculitides, it does play a role in its treatment and has been met with success in specific case studies [62, 67].

Dosage and Side Effects

Once methotrexate is absorbed, it undergoes a triphasic reduction. The first phase occurs within 75 min of ingestion and relates to systemic distribution throughout the body. The second phase lasting 2–4 h represents renal excretion. Lastly, the third phase can last between 10 and 27 h, being especially long because it corresponds with the slow release of methotrexate from DHFR in tissues [68]. While ~50% of methotrexate is plasma bound, its toxicity lies in the remaining amount that is found unbound [8]. Factors that may influence its toxicity may be prolonged drug clearance (renal insufficiency) time, as well as displacement from plasma proteins by other drugs (increasing plasma methotrexate concentrations). Methotrexate is minimally metabolized throughout the body; 50–90% is excreted unchanged in the urine [7]. Drug accumulation in the liver and kidney can occur at high doses and over prolonged periods of therapy. Ultimately, this may play an important role in toxicity [59].

Bone marrow suppression is the major dose-limiting factor when administering methotrexate therapy [69]. Methotrexate-induced hepatotoxcity may also occur during short- or long-term use. Chronically, this may lead to hepatic fibrosis and, rarely, cirrhosis [59]. Pulmonary toxicity manifested as acute pneumonitis or pulmonary fibrosis may also occur in this patient population. Resolution usually occurs after discontinuation of therapy. The cause of pneumonitis is thought to be an idiosyncratic reaction or a hypersensitivity reaction [70].

Gastrointestinal toxicity commonly occurs and is dose dependent. This may manifest as nausea, ulcerative mucositis, and diarrhea [71]. Other side effects include renal failure, alopecia, dermatitis, photophobia, increased ocular discomfort and epiphora [29, 59] (see table 5).

Table 5. Special considerations for methotrexate

Contraindications to treatment • Decreased renal and liver function, especially in the elderly • Alcoholics, alcoholic liver disease, or known active hepatic disease • Hypersensitivity to drug • Pregnancy class X • Excreted in breast milk
Drug interactions • Drugs that displace methotrexate from plasma proteins may increase systemic concentrations (e.g. consumption of salicylates, sulfonamides, chloramphenicol, tetracycline) • Drugs that decrease renal blood flow or tubular secretion may increase systemic concentrations (e.g. NSAIDs or probenecid)

Systemic Immunosuppressive Therapy for Eye Disease Study

Methotrexate was not found to be associated significantly with an increase in the incidence of mortality (fully adjusted hazard ratio: 1.02, 95% CI 0.78–1.34) or cancer-related mortality (fully adjusted hazard ratio: 0.89, 95% CI 0.48–1.63) [50, 51]. These findings are well supported in the literature by multiple studies in patients who have received chronic treatment with methotrexate for psoriasis and rheumatoid arthritis [72–76].

Azathioprine

History and Source

Azathioprine was first developed in the 1960s for the use of immunosuppression in transplant patients, and in the treatment of autoimmune diseases [25]. By 1966, Newell began using it to treat ocular immune-mediated disorders [77, 78].

Pharmacology

This prodrug is metabolized in the liver to its active metabolite 6-mercatopurine. As 6-mercaptopurine is converted to thionosine-5-phosphate (a purine analog), it is able to act as false precursor to the formation of purine nucleotides, thus, inhibiting the formation of adenine and guanine. This results in impaired DNA synthesis, RNA synthesis, and protein synthesis [7].

Clinical Pharmacology

At the normally prescribed dose, 2–3 mg/kg, azathioprine strongly suppresses T cells, but weakly suppresses B cells [79]. In addition, it depresses the formation of monocyte precursors [8]. At larger doses, alteration in antibody response may be elicited [79].

Therapeutic Effects
Azathioprine has been shown to be effective in the treatment of various corticosteroid-resistant ocular inflammatory diseases. In particular, the literature notes its efficacy for the treatment of scleritis associated with polychondritis, ocular cicatricial pemphigoid, pars planitis, and JIA-associated iridocyclitis [20, 66, 78, 80]. In a 2-year double-masked, randomized, controlled study, it was demonstrated that azathioprine (2.5 mg/kg/day) was able to prevent the formation of new eye lesions and reduce the frequency and intensity of inflammation in patients with ABD [81]. However, Foster found more equivocal efficacy in a series of 8 patients treated similarly [82]. There has also been varying results for its use in the treatment of sympathetic ophthalmia [24, 78].

Dosage and Side Effects
Once ingested orally, within 2 h 50% is absorbed [25]. From there, it is metabolized in erythrocytes and in the liver to its active form, 6-MP. Approximately 30% of 6-MP is maintained bound by plasma proteins. Renal clearance accounts for only 2% of drug excretion; however, there is increased cytotoxicity in patients with renal insufficiency [25].

Myelosuppression is a common side effect of azathioprine often occurring as a delayed response to treatment, following 1–2 weeks after beginning therapy [1]. The most common side effects experienced by patients on this therapy are gastrointestinal upset, nausea, vomiting, and diarrhea. Often, these symptoms become the reason for discontinuation of this drug [81]. Other known side effects, albeit less common, include interstitial pneumonitis, hepatocellular necrosis, pancreatitis, stomatitis, alopecia, and (rarely) secondary infections [83, 84] (see table 6).

Systemic Immunosuppressive Therapy for Eye Disease Study
Azathioprine was not found to be significantly associated with an increase in the incidence of mortality (fully adjusted hazard ratio: 0.99, 95% CI 0.72–1.38) or cancer-related mortality (fully adjusted hazard ratio: 1.13, 95% CI 0.60–2.14) [50, 51]. Multiple previous studies support these findings in patients who have been treated with azathioprine chronically for rheumatoid arthritis and inflammatory bowel disease [85–89].

Antibiotics

Cyclosporine

History and Source
In the early 1970s, cyclosporin A (CSA) was discovered by the researchers at Sandoz laboratories [90, 91]. It was derived from cultures of the fungi *Tolypocladium inflatum*. The effectiveness of CSA for the treatment of autoimmune uveitis was first reported by Nussenblatt et al. [92, 93] in 1983.

Table 6. Special considerations for azathioprine

Contraindications to treatment • Patients with renal impairment • Hypersensitivity to the drug • Immunosuppressed patients with rheumatoid arthritis previously treated with alkylating agent in whom the risk of the development of neoplasia is potentially high • Pregnancy class D • Excreted in breast milk in low concentration
Drug interactions • Allopurinol (inhibits xanthine oxidase, thus impairing conversion of azathioprine to its metabolite; reduce dose by 25%) • Severe leukopenia associated with ACE inhibitors • The metabolism of azathioprine is affected by drugs that interact with the P-450 mixed function oxidase system • Mutations in the methyltransferase gene may lead to increased concentrations of active 6-mercaptopurine and increased drug toxicity

Pharmacology

CSA reversibly inhibits T cell-mediated alloimmune and autoimmune responses. It is believed that CSA disrupts the transmission of signals from the T cell receptor to the genes that specifically encode for the lymphokines and enzymes, responsible for activating resting T cells and cytoaggression, while leaving the T cell priming reaction unaffected [94, 95].

Clinical Pharmacology

The production of specific proinflammatory factors in the T cell are potentiated through a series of Ca^{+}-dependent pathways. CSA acts intracellularly to form a ternary complex with calcineurin, thus inhibiting this Ca^{+}-dependent pathway. This calcineurin complex leads to inhibition of calmodulin binding with Ca^{+2}-activated phosphatase activity of calcineurin. In turn, this leads to inhibition of the dephosphorylation of the cytoplasmic subunit of nuclear factor of activated T cells (NF-AT). The proper functioning of NF-AT is crucial in the activation of transcription of specific cellular immune signals. In particular, IL-2, IL-3, IL-4, IL-5, TNF-c, and interferon-γ [96–99]. CSA acts most specifically to inhibit T helper cells while leaving T suppressor cells active. Thus, the overall result is a marked reduction in antibody production to T cell-dependent antigens and an inhibition of T cell cytotoxic activity [83].

Therapeutic Value

Nussenblatt and coworkers were the first to provide positive report in favor of treating patients with poorly controllable uveitis with CSA. At doses of 10 mg/kg/day, it was found that uveitis may be controlled in ABD, birdshot retinochoroidopathy, sarcoidosis, pars planitis, Vogt-Koyanagi-Harada (VKH), MS, sympathetic ophthalmia, and idiopathic vitritis [92, 93, 100–102]. These findings were supported by other investigators in two uncontrolled, nonrandomized trials, and in the treatment of birdshot retinochoroidopathy, ABD, and VKH [102–106]. In a more recent randomized double-masked trial by Nussenblatt et al. [107], CSA was shown to be effective in the treatment of intraocular inflammation in 46% of patients intolerant to corticosteroids; additionally, another 35% responded to combination therapy with corticosteroids. Two additional randomized double-masked trials corroborated its effectiveness as an effective anti-inflammatory medication [108, 109]. However, in these studies, CSA was prescribed at 10 mg/kg/day; a dose that is now known to be highly nephrotoxic and hypertensive. Lower doses of CSA at 4 mg/kg/day and then 2.5 mg/kg/day were later tried in hopes of achieving similar anti-inflammatory results and with less toxicity [110–113]. It has been shown that at lower doses 5–7.5 mg/kg/day, CSA is inferior for the treatment of ABD in comparison to other IMTs (chlorambucil, cyclophosphamide, and azathioprine) [82, 114]. Other areas of potential efficacy are in patients who are at high risk for corneal transplant rejection, and in patients with corneal ulceration associated with granulomatosis with polyangiitis and peripheral ulcerative keratitis, as well as ligneous conjunctivitis, and vernal conjunctivitis [115–125].

Dosage and Side Effects

When administered orally, the absorption of this medication in the gastrointestinal tract can be quite variable. The mean bioavailability is 30% of the original dose [126]. The drug should be ingested with food so as to increase its absorption [26]. Initially, when CSA is absorbed into the blood stream, 90% is found bound to plasma proteins. Ultimately, 60–75% of the drug becomes transported into erythrocytes, and 10–20% into leukocytes [126]. In patients with chronic flare, it has been found that the concentration in the aqueous of CSA is 40% that of the plasma concentration [127]. CSA is metabolized in the liver by the hepatic microsomal cytochrome P-450 mixed function oxidase system. Enterohepatic recirculation occurs with most of the drug excreted in the bile and 6% in the urine. Like other drugs dependent on the cytochrome P-450, liver function and co-interaction with other drugs can be significant to CSA clearance.

The original dosing of CSA at 10 mg/kg/day was fraught with serious complications, in particular renal impairment and HTN [128]. These complications are dose specific, and seen at a much lower frequency with the doses that are currently employed (2.5–5 mg/kg/day) [113, 129]. Furthermore, with careful monitoring of BUN and creatinine clearance, any significant change in renal function can often be reversible if attended to in a timely manner by either discontinuing treatment or decreasing the dosage. It has been suggested that at doses of 5 mg/kg/day, permanent renal damage can be avoided if the serum creatinine value remains within 30% of its baseline value [130]. Similarly, HTN is reversible and dose dependent. At doses of <5 mg/kg/day, HTN is observed in ~15–27% of patients [131, 132] Other laboratory findings to

Table 7. Special considerations for cyclosporine

Contraindications to treatment • Patients with a past medical history of uncontrolled systemic hypertension, hepatic disease, and renal insufficiency • Hypersensitivity to the drug • Pregnancy class C • Excreted in breast milk
Drug interactions • Drugs that inhibit renal flow may potentiate its nephrotoxic effects (e.g. aminoglycosides, amphotericin B, ketaconazole, vancomycin, melphalan, cimetidine, ranitidine, trimethoprim with sulfamethoxazole, ciprofloxacin, and NSAIDs) • The metabolism of CSA is affected by drugs that interact with the P-450 mixed function oxidase system
Dietary considerations • CSA can cause retention of potassium • CSA can cause hypomagnesemia • Omega-3 may help to reduce blood pressure • Food increases the absorption of CSA • Grapefruit juice can cause significant rise in drug blood levels

note while on CSA therapy is an association with normochromic, normocytic anemia (25%) and an increased ESR (40%), and mild changes in serum transaminases and bilirubin levels [133, 134].

Other adverse reactions that occur frequently are paresthesias or burning sensation (70%), fatigue (67%), headache (57%) nausea (43%), hirsuitism (50–57%), gingival hyperplasia (25–43%), tremor (38%), increased risk of opportunistic infections (38%), visual acuity changes, and visual hallucinations [29, 35, 83, 84,132, 135, 136] (see table 7).

Systemic Immunosuppressive Therapy for Eye Disease Study
Cyclosporine was not found to be significantly associated with an increase in the incidence of mortality (fully adjusted hazard ratio: 0.79, 95% CI 0.57–1.10) or cancer-related mortality (fully adjusted hazard ratio: 0.82, 95% CI 0.40–1.67) [50, 51]. These findings are in agreement with other retrospective studies done on patients receiving chronic CSA therapy, either for rheumatoid arthritis or psoriasis (although this study did note increased incidence of skin cancers) [33, 137, 138].

Major Reactions & Interactions

For an overview of the major adverse reactions and the interactions with the drugs to be discussed in this chapter, see Tables 8 and 9.

Table 8. Major adverse reactions to conventional immunosuppressive drugs

Drug	Adverse reaction
Cyclophosphamide	sterile hemorrhagic cystitis, myelosuppression, gonadal dysfunction, secondary malignancies, pulmonary fibrosis
Chlorambucil	sterile hemorrhagic cystitis, myelosuppression, gonadal dysfunction, secondary malignancies, pulmonary fibrosis
Methotrexate	myelosuppression, hepatotoxicity, pneumonitis, ulcerative stomatitis, diarrhea
Azathioprine	myelosuppression, hepatotoxicity, pneumonitis, ulcerative stomatitis, diarrhea
CSA	nephrotoxicity, hypertension, hepatotoxicity, hyperuricemia, hyperglycemia, nausea and vomiting

Table 9. Drugs that interact with the P-450 mixed function oxidase system

Inhibitors Protease inhibitors, clarithromycin, erythromycin, chloramphenicol, ciprofloxacin, ketaconazole, itraconazole, fluconazole, voriconazole, verapamil, dilitiazem, amiodarone, bergamottin (constituent of grapefruit juice), fluoxetine, paroxetine, cimetidine
Inducers Carbamazepine, phenytoin, oxcarbazepine, phenobarbital, ethanol, isoniazid, St. John's wort, rifampicin, rifabutin, non-nucleoside reverse transcriptase inhibitors, pioglitazone, troglitazone, glucocorticoids, modafinil

References

1 Dorr R, Fritz W: Cancer Chemotherapy Handbook. Amsterdam, Elsevier, 1980.

2 Krumbhaar EB, Krumbhaar HD: The blood and bone marrow in yellow cross gas (mustard gas) poisoning: changes produced in the bone marrow of fatal cases. J Med Res 1919;40:497–507.

3 Gery I, Nussenblatt RB: Immunosuppressive drugs; in Sears ML (eds): Pharmacology of the Eye. Berlin, Springer, 1984, pp 586–609.

4 Roda-Perez E: Sobre un case se uveitis de etiologia ignota tratado con mostaza introgenada. Rev Clin Esp 1951;40:265–267.

5 Roda-Perez E: El tratamiento de las uveitis de etiologia ignota con mostaza nitrogenada. Arch Soc Ofial Hisp Am 1952;12:131–151.

6 Brock N: Oxazaphosphorine cytostatics: past-present-future: Seventh Cain Memorial Award Lecture. Cancer Res 1989;49:1–7.

7 Calabresi P, Chabner BA: Chemotherapy of neoplastic diseases; in Gilman AG, Rall TW, Nies AS, Taylor P (eds): Goodman and Gilman's the Pharmacological Basis of Therapeutics. New York, Pergamon Press, 1990, pp 1202–1263.

8 Foster CS: Pharmacologic treatment of immune disorders; in Albert DM, Jakobiec FA (eds): Principles and Practice of Ophthalmology, Basic Sciences. Philadelphia, WB Saunders, 1994, pp 1076–1084.

9 Stockman GP, Heim LR, South MA, Trentin JJ: Differential effects of cyclophosphamide on the B and T cell compartments of adult mice. J Immunol 1973;110:277–282.

10 Clements PJ, Yu DTY, Levy J, Paulus HE, Barnett EU: Effects of cyclophosphamide on B and T lymphocytes in rheumatoid arthritis. Arthritis Rheum 1974;17:347–353.

11 Fauci AS, Date DC, Wolff SM: Cyclophosphamide and lymphocyte subpopulations in Wegener's granulomatosis. Arthritis Rheum 1974;17:355–361.

12 Lerman SP, Weidanz WP: The effect of cyclophosphamide on the ontogeny of the humoral immune response in chickens. J Immunol 1970;105:614–619.

13 Hemady R, Tauber J, Foster CS: Immunosuppressive drugs in immune and inflammatory disease. Surv Ophthalmol 1991:35:359–385.

14 Brubaker R, Font RL, Shepero EM: Granulomatous sclerouveitis, regression of ocular lesions with cyclophosphamide and prednisone. Arch Ophthalmol 1971;86:517–524.
15 Foster CS: Immunosuppressive therapy for external ocular inflammatory disease. Ophthalmology 1980; 87:140–150.
16 Jampol LM, West C, Goldberg MF: Therapy of scleritis with cytotoxic agents. Am J Ophthalmol 1978;86:266–271.
17 Fauci AS, Haynes BF, Katz P, Wolff SM: Wegener's granulomatosis: prospective clinical and therapeutic experience with 85 patients for 21 years. Ann Intern Med 1983;98:75–85.
18 Foster CS: Systemic immunosuppressive therapy for progressive bilateral Mooren's ulcer. Ophthalmology 1985,92:1436–1439.
19 Brown SI, Mondino BJ: Therapy of Mooren's ulcer. Am J Ophthalmol 1984;98:1–6.
20 Foster CS: Cicatricial pemphigoid. Trans Am Ophthalmol Soc 1986;84:527–663.
21 Oniki S, Kurakazu K, Kawata K: Immunosuppressive treatment of Behcet's disease with cyclophosphamide. Jpn J Ophthalmol 1976;20:32–40.
22 Fain O, Du LTH, Wechsler B: Pulse cyclophosphamide in Behçet's disease; in: O'Duffy JD, Kokmen E (eds): Behçet's Disease: Basic and Clinical Aspects. New York: Marcel Dekker, 1991, pp 569–573.
23 Buckley CE, Durham NC, Gills JP: Cyclophosphamide therapy of peripheral uveitis. Arch Intern Med 1969;124:29–35.
24 Martenet AC: Immunosuppressive therapy of uveitis: mid- and long-term follow up after classical cytostatic treatment; in Usui M, Ohno S, Aoki K (eds): Ocular Immunology Today. New York: Excerpta Medica, 1990, pp 443–446.
25 Rapini RP, Jordan RE, Wolverton SE: Cytotoxic agents; in Wolverton SE, Wilkins JK (eds): Systemic Drugs for Skin Diseases. Philadelphia: WB Saunders, 1991, pp 125–151.
26 AMA drug evaluations. Chicago, American Medical Association, 1991, pp 396, 1059, 1654–1655, 1671–1672, 1843–1844, 1972–1973, 1891–1913, 2009–2034, 2140–2141, 2351–2353.
27 Fairley KF, Barrie JV, Johnson W: Sterility and testicular atrophy related to cyclophosphamide therapy. Lancet 1972;1:568–569.
28 Berkson BM, Come LG, Shapiro I: Severe cystitis induced by cyclophosphamide, role of surgical management. JAMA 1973;225:605–606.
29 Fraunfelder FT, Meyer SM: Ocular toxicity from antineoplastic agents. Ophthalmology 1983;90:1–3.
30 Puri HC, Campbell RA: Cyclophosphamide and malignancy. Lancet 1977;1:1306.
31 Baker GL, Kahl LE, Zee BC, Stolzer BL, Agarwal AK, Medsger TA Jr: Malignancy following treatment of rheumatoid arthritis with cyclophosphamide. Long-term case-control follow-up study. Am J Med 1987;83:1–9.
32 Baltus JA, Boersma JW, Hartman AP, Vandenbroucke JP: The occurrence of malignancies in patients with rheumatoid arthritis treated with cyclophosphamide: a controlled retrospective follow-up. Ann Rheum Dis 1983;42:368–373.
33 Kempen JH, Gangaputra S, Daniel E, Levy-Clarke GA, Nussenblatt RB, Rosenbaum JT: Long-term risk of malignancy among patients treated with immunosuppressive agents for ocular inflammation: a critical assessment of the evidence. Am J Ophthalmol 2008;146:802–812.
34 Mamo JG, Azzam SA: Treatment of Behcet's disease with chlorambucil. Arch Ophthalmol 1970;84: 446–450.
35 Rubin B, Palestine AG: Complications of corticosteroids and immunosuppressive drugs. Int Ophthalmol Clin 1989;29:159–169.
36 Ben Ezra D, Cohen E: Treatment and visual prognosis in Behcet's disease. Br J Ophthalmol 1986;70:589–592.
37 Bietti GB, Ceruili L, Pivetti-Pezzi P: Behcet's disease and immunosuppressive treatment. Mod Probl Ophthalmol 1976;16:314–323.
38 O'Duffy JD, Robertson DM, Goldstein NP: Chlorambucil in the treatment of uveitis and meningoencephalitis of Behcet's disease. Am J Med 1984;76:75–84.
39 Pezzi PD, Gaspani U, DeLiso P, Catarinelli G: Prognosis in Behcet's disease. Ann Ophthalmol 1985;17:20–25.
40 Tricoulis D: Treatment of Behcet's disease with chlorambucil. Br J Ophthalmol 1976;60:55–57.
41 Abdalla MI, Bahgat N: Long-lasting remission of Behcet's disease after chlorambucil therapy. Br J Ophthalmol 1993;57:706–710.
42 Elliot JH, Ballinger WH: Behcet's syndrome. Treatment with chlorambucil. Trans Am Ophthalmol Soc 1984;82:264–281.
43 Godfrey WA, Epstein WV, O'Connor GR, et al: The use of chlorambucil in intractable idiopathic uveitis. Am J Ophthalmol 1974;78:415–428.
44 Kanski JJ: Anterior uveitis in juvenile rheumatoid arthritis. Arch Ophthalmol 1977;95:1794–1797.
45 Foster CS, Barrett F: Cataract development and cataract surgery in patients with juvenile rheumatoid arthritis-associated iridocyclitis. Ophthalmology 1993;100:809–817.
46 Jennings T, Tessler HH: Twenty cases of sympathetic ophthalmia. Br J Ophthalmol 1989;73:140–145.
47 Clements PJ, Davis J: Cytotoxic drugs: Their clinical application to the rheumatic diseases. Semin Arthritis Rheum 1986;15:231–254.

48 Tabbara KF: Chlorambucil in Behcet's disease, a reappraisal. Ophthalmology 1983;90:906–908.
49 Williams SA, Makker SP, Grupe WE: Seizures, a significant side effect of chlorambucil therapy in children. J Pediatr 1978;93:510–518.
50 Kempen JH, Daniel E, Dunn JP, Foster CS, Gangaputra S, Hanish A, Helzlsouer KJ, Jabs DA, Kaçmaz RO, Levy-Clarke GA, Liesegang TL, Newcomb CW, Nussenblatt RB, Pujari SS, Rosenbaum JT, Suhler EB, Thorne JE: Overall and cancer related mortality among patients with ocular inflammation treated with immunosuppressive drugs: retrospective cohort study. BMJ 2009;339:b2480.
51 Kempen JH, Daniel E, Gangaputra S, Dreger K, Jabs DA, Kacmaz RO: Methods for identifying long-term adverse effects of treatment in patients with eye diseases: the Systemic Immunosuppressive Therapy for Eye Diseases (SITE) cohort study. Ophthalmic Epidemiol 2008;15:47–55.
52 Berk PA, Goldberg JD, Silverman MN, et al: Increased incidence of acute leukemia in polycythemia vera associated with chlorambucil therapy. N Engl J Med 1981;304:441–447.
53 Lemer HJ: Acute myelogenous leukemia in students receiving chlorambucil as long-term adjuvant chemotherapy for stage II breast cancer. Cancer Treat Rep 1978;62:1135–1138.
54 Smith AL (ed): Oxford Dictionary of Biochemistry and Molecular Biology. Oxford: Oxford University Press, pp 43.
55 Farber S, Diamond LK, Mercer RD: Temporary remissions in acute leukemia in children produced by folic antagonist 4-amethopteroylglutamic acid (aminopterin). N Engl J Med 1948;238:787–793.
56 Weinblatt ME, Kremer JM: Methotrexate in rheumatoid arthritis. J Am Acad Dermatol 1988;19: 126–128.
57 Lally EV, Ho G: A review of methotrexate therapy in Reiter's syndrome. Semin Arthritis Rheum 1985;15: 139–145.
58 Wong VG, Hersh EM: Methotrexate in the therapy of cyclitis. Trans Am Acad Ophthalmol Otolaryngol 1965;69:279–293.
59 Callen JP, Kulp-Shorten CL: Methotrexate; in Wolverton SE, Wilkins JK (eds): Systemic Drugs for Skin Diseases. Philadelphia: WB Saunders, 1991, pp 152–166.
60 Andersen PA, West SG, O'Dell JR: Weekly pulse methotrexate in rheumatoid arthritis. Clinical and immunologic effects in a randomized, double-blind study. Ann Intern Med 1985;103:489–496.
61 Weinblatt ME, Coblyn JS, Fox DA: Efficacy of low-dose methotrexate in rheumatoid arthritis. N Engl J Med 1985;312:818–822.
62 Shah SS, Lowder CY, Schmidt MA, et al: Low-dose methotrexate therapy for ocular inflammatory disease. Ophthalmology 1992;99:1419–1423.
63 Wong VG: Methotrexate treatment of uveal disease. Am J Med Sci 1966;251:239–241.
64 Wong VG, Hersh EM, McMaster PRB: Treatment of a presumed case of sympathetic ophthalmia with methotrexate. Arch Ophthalmol 1966;76:66–76.
65 Walker AM, Funch D, Dreyer NA: Determinants of serious liver disease among patients receiving low-dose methotrexate for rheumatoid arthritis. Arthritis Rheum 1993;36:329–335.
66 Huang-Xuan T, Foster CS, Rice BA: Scleritis in relapsing polychondritis: response to therapy. Ophthalmology 1990;97:892–898.
67 Dev S, McCallum RM, Jaffee GJ: Methotrexate treatment for sarcoid-associated panuveitis. Ophthalmology 1999;106:111.
68 Olsen EA: The pharmacology of methotrexate. J Am Acad Dermatol 1991;25:306–317.
69 Shupack JL, Webster OF: Pancytopenia following low-dose oral methotrexate therapy for psoriasis. JAMA 1988;259:3594–3596.
70 Ridley MG, Wolfe CS, Mathews JH: Life-threatening acute pneumonitis during low-dose methotrexate treatment for rheumatoid arthritis: a case report and review of the literature. Ann Rheum Dis 1988; 47:784–788.
71 Schein PS, Winokur SH: Immunosuppressive and cytotoxic chemotherapy: long-term complications. Ann Intern Med 1975;82:94–95.
72 Bailin PL, Tindall JP, Roenigk HH Jr, Hogan MD: Is methotrexate therapy for psoriasis carcinogenic? A modified retrospective-prospective analysis. JAMA 1975;232:359–362.
73 Nyfors A, Jensen H: Frequency of malignant neoplasms in 248 long-term methotrexate-treated psoriatics. A preliminary study. Dermatologica 1983; 167:260–261.
74 Wolfe F, Michaud K: The effect of methotrexate and anti-tumor necrosis factor therapy on the risk of lymphoma in rheumatoid arthritis in 19,562 patients during 89,710 person-years of observation. Arthritis Rheum 2007;56:1433–1439.
75 Tishler M, Caspi D, Yaron M: Long-term experience with low-dose methotrexate in rheumatoid arthritis. Rheumatol Int 1993;13:103–106.
76 Georgescu L, Quinn GC, Schwartzman S, Paget SA: Lymphoma in patients with rheumatoid arthritis: association with the disease state or methotrexate treatment. Semin Arthritis Rheum 1997;26:794–804.
77 Newell FW, Krill AE: Treatment of uveitis with azathioprine (Imuran). Trans Ophthalmol Soc UK 1967;87:499–511.

78 Newell FW, Krill AE, Thompson A: The treatment of uveitis with six-mercaptopurine. Am J Ophthalmol 1966;61:1250–1255.
79 Bach JH: The Mode of Action of Immunosuppressive Drugs. Amsterdam, Elsevier, 1975.
80 Hemady R, Baer JC, Foster CS: Immunosuppressive drugs in the management of progressive, corticosteroid-resistant uveitis associated with juvenile rheumatoid arthritis. Int Ophthalmol Clin 1992;32:241–252.
81 Yazici H, Pazarli H, Bames CG: A controlled trial of azathioprine in Behcet's syndrome. N Engl J Med 1990;322:281–285.
82 Foster CS, Baer JC, Raizman MB: Therapeutic responses to systemic immunosuppressive chemotherapy agents in patients with Behcet's syndrome affecting the eyes; in O'Duffy JD, Kokmen E (eds): Behcet's Disease: Basic and Clinical Aspects. New York: Marcel Dekker, 1991, pp 581–588.
83 Pavan-Langston D, Dunkel EC: Handbook of Ocular Drug Therapy and Ocular Side Effects of Systemic Drugs. Boston, Little, Brown, 1991, pp 203–213.
84 Nussenblatt RB, Palestine AG: Uveitis, Fundamentals and Clinical Practice. Chicago: Year Book Medical Publishers, 1989, pp 116–144.
85 Singh G, Fries JF, Spitz P, Williams CA: Toxic effects of azathioprine in rheumatoid arthritis. A national post-marketing perspective. Arthritis Rheum 1989; 32:837–843.
86 Castor CW, Bull FE: Review of United States data on neoplasms in rheumatoid arthritis. Am J Med 1985; 78:33–38.
87 Hazleman BL: The comparative incidence of malignant disease in rheumatoid arthritics exposed to different treatment regimens. Ann Rheum Dis 1982;41:12–17.
88 Fraser AG, Orchard TR, Robinson EM, Jewell DP: Long-term risk of malignancy after treatment of inflammatory bowel disease with azathioprine. Aliment Pharmacol Ther 2002;16:1225–1232.
89 Connell WR, Kamm MA, Dickson M, Balkwill AM, Ritchie JK, Lennard-Jones JE: Long-term neoplasia risk after azathioprine treatment in inflammatory bowel disease. Lancet 1994;343:1249–1252.
90 Borel JF: The history of cyclosporin A and its significance; White DJG (eds): Cyclosporin A. New York: Elsevier, 1982, pp 5–17.
91 Heusler K, Pletscher A: The controversial early history of cyclosporine. Swiss Med Wkly 2001;131:299–302.
92 Nussenblatt RB, Palestine AG, Rook AH: Treatment of intraocular inflammation with cyclosporin A. Lancet 1983;1:235–238.
93 Nussenblatt RB, Palestine AG, Chan CC: Cyclosporine A therapy in the treatment of intraocular inflammatory disease resistant to systemic corticosteroids and cytotoxic agents. Am J Ophthalmol 1983;96:275–282.
94 deSmet MD, Nussenblatt RB: Clinical use of cyclosporine in ocular disease. Int Ophthalmol Clin 1993;33:31–45.
95 Sigal NH, Dumont FJ: Cyclosporin A, FK-506, and rapamycin: pharmacologic probes of lymphocyte signal transduction. Annu Rev Immunol 1992;10: 519–560.
96 Liu J: FK 506 and cyclosporin, molecular probes for studying intracellular signal transduction. Immunol Today 1993;14:290–295.
97 Sigal SN: Immunosuppressive profile of rapamycin. Ann N Y Acad Sci 1993;685:1–8.
98 Chang JY, Sehgal SN: Pharmacology of rapamycin: a new immunosuppressive agent. B J Rheumatol 1991;30(suppl 2):62–65.
99 Chang JY, Sehgal SN, Bansbach CC: FK 506 and rapamycin: novel pharmacological probes of the immune response. Trends Pharmacol Sci 1991;12: 218–223.
100 Nussenblatt RB, Palestine AG, Chan CC, Ochizuki M, Yancey K: Effectiveness of cyclosporine therapy for Behcet's disease. Arthritis Rheum 1985;28:671–679.
101 Nussenblatt RB, Palestine AG, Chan CC: Improvement of uveitis and optic nerve disease by cyclosporine in a patient with multiple sclerosis. Am J Ophthalmol 1984;97:790–791.
102 Nussenblatt RB, Palestine AG, Chan CC: Cyclosporine therapy for uveitis: long-term follow up. J Ocul Pharmacol 1985;1:369–382.
103 Graham EM, Sanders MD, James DG, et al: Cyclosporin A in the treatment of posterior uveitis. Trans Ophthalmol Soc UK 1985;104:146–151.
104 LeHoang P, Girard B, Deray G: Cyclosporine in the treatment of birdshot retinochoroidopathy. Transplant Proc 1988;20(suppl 4):128–130.
105 Binder Al, Graham EM, Sanders MD: Cyclosporin A in the treatment of severe Behcet's uveitis. Br J Rheumatol 1987;76:285–291.
106 Wakefield D, McCluskey P, Reece G: Cyclosporin therapy in Vogt-Koyanagi-Harada disease. Aust N Z J Ophthalmol 1990;18:137–142.
107 Nussenblatt RB, Palestine AG, Chan CC: Randomized, double-masked study of cyclosporine compared to prednisolone in the treatment of endogenous uveitis. Am J Ophthalmol 1991;112:38–146.
108 Masuda K, Nakajima A, Urayama A: Double-masked trial of cyclosporin versus colchicine and long-term open study of cyclosporine in Behcet's disease. Lancet 1989;1:1093–1096.
109 deVries J, Baarsma GS, Zaai MJW: Cyclosporin in the treatment of severe chronic idiopathic uveitis. Br J Ophthalmol 1990;74:344–349.
110 Towler HMA, Cliffe AM, Whiting PH, Forrester JV: Low dose cyclosporin A therapy in chronic posterior uveitis. Eye 1989;3:282–287.

111 Towler HMA, Whiting PH, Forrester JV: Combination low dose cyclosporin A and steroid therapy in chronic intraocular inflammation. Eye 1990;4: 514–520.

112 Towler HMA, Lightman SL, Forrester JV: Low-dose cyclosporine therapy of ocular inflammation: preliminary report of a long-term follow-up study. J Autoimmun 1992;5(suppl A):259–264.

113 Vitale AT, Rodriguez A, Foster CS: Low-dose cyclosporine therapy in the treatment of birdshot retinochoroidopathy. Ophthalmology 1994;101:782–831.

114 Chavis PS, Antonios SR, Tabbara KF: Cyclosporine effects on optic nerve and retinal vasculitis in Behcet's disease. Doc Ophthalmol 1992;80:133–142.

115 Hill JC: The use of cyclosporine in high-risk keratoplasty. Am J Ophthalmol 1989;107:506–510.

116 Miller K, Huber C, Niederwieser D, Gottinger W: Successful engraftment of high-risk corneal allografts with short-term immunosuppression with cyclosporine. Transplantation 1988;45:651–653.

117 Hoffman F, Widerholt M: Local treatment of necrotizing scleritis with cyclosporin A. Cornea 1985;4: 3–7.

118 Wiebking WJ, Mehlfeld T: Local treatment of corneal ulcers and scleromalacias with cyclosporin A. Fortschr Ophthalmol 1986;83:345–347.

119 Kruit PJ, VanBalen AT, Stilma JS: Cyclosporin A treatment in two cases of corneal peripheral melting syndromes. Doc Ophthalmol 1985;59:33–39.

120 Kruit PJ: Cyclosporine A treatment in four cases with corneal melting syndrome. Transplant Proc 1988;90(suppl):170–172.

121 Holland EJ, Chan CC, Kuwabara T: Immunohistological findings and results of treatment with cyclosporine in ligneous conjunctivitis. Am J Ophthalmol 1989;107:160–166.

122 Rubin BI, Holland EJ, deSmet MD: Response of reactivated ligneous conjunctivitis to topical cyclosporine. Am J Ophthalmol 1991;112:95–96.

123 Ben Ezra D, Peter J, Brodsky M, Cohen E: Cyclosporine eyedrops for the treatment of severe vernal keratoconjunctivitis. Am J Ophthalmol 1986;101: 278–282.

124 Bleik PH, Tabbara KF: Topical cyclosporine in vernal keratoconjunctivitis. Ophthalmology 1991;98: 1679–1684.

125 Secchi AG, Tognon MS, Leonardi A: Topical use of cyclosporine in the treatment of vernal keratoconjunctivitis. Am J Ophthalmol 1990;110:641–645.

126 Handschumacher RE: Immunosuppressive agents; in Gilman AC, Rail TW, Nies AS, Taylor P (eds): Goodman and Gilman's The Pharmacological Basis of Therapeutics. New York: Pergamon Press, 1990, pp 1264–1276.

127 Palestine AG, Nussenblatt RE, Chan CC: Cyclosporine penetration into the anterior chamber and cerebrospinal fluid. Am J Ophthalmol 1985;99:210–211.

128 Kahan BD: Cyclosporine nephrotoxicity: pathogenesis, prophylaxis, therapy and prognosis. Am J Kidney Dis 1986;8:323–331.

129 Nussenblatt RB, de Smet MD, Rubin B: A masked, randomized, dose-response study between cyclosporine A and G in the treatment of sight-threatening uveitis of noninfectious origin. Am J Ophthalmol 1993;115:583–591.

130 Feutren G, Mihatsch MJ: Risk factors for cyclosporine-induced nephrotoxicity in patients with autoimmune diseases. N Engl J Med 1992;326:1654–1660.

131 de Groen PL: Cyclosporine. A review and its specific use in liver transplantation. Mayo Clin Proc 1989;64:680–689.

132 Mathews D, Mathews J, Jones NP: Low-dose cyclosporine treatment for sight-threatening uveitis: efficacy, toxicity, and tolerance. Indian J Ophthalmol 2010;58:55–58.

133 Palestine AG, Nussenblatt RB, Chan CC: Side effects of systemic cyclosporine in patients not undergoing transplantation. Am J Med 1984;77:652–656.

134 Kahan BD: Cyclosporine. N Engl J Med 1989;321: 1725–1738.

135 Nussenblatt RB, Palestine AG: Cyclosporine: immunology, pharmacology and therapeutic uses. Surv Ophthalmol 1986;31:159–169.

136 Foster CS: Nonsteroidal anti-inflammatory and immunosuppressive agents; in Lamberts DW, Potter DE (eds): Clinical Ophthalmic Pharmacology. Boston, Little, Brown, 1987, pp 181–192.

137 Van den Borne BE, Landewe RB, Houkes I, Schild F, van der Heyden PC, Hazes JM: No increased risk of malignancies and mortality in cyclosporin A-treated patients with rheumatoid arthritis. Arthritis Rheum 1998;41:1930–1937.

138 Paul CF, Ho VC, McGeown C, Christophers E, Schmidtmann B, Guillaume JC: Risk of malignancies in psoriasis patients treated with cyclosporine: a 5 y cohort study. J Invest Dermatol 2003;120:211–216.

Jonathan Kruh, MD
Massachusetts Eye Research and Surgery Institution
Ocular Immunology and Uveitis Foundation
5 Cambridge Center, 8th Floor
Cambridge, MA 02142 (USA)
Tel. +1 617 621 6377, E-Mail jkruh@mersi.com

Miserocchi E, Modorati G, Foster CS (eds): New Treatments in Noninfectious Uveitis.
Dev Ophthalmol. Basel, Karger, 2012, vol 51, pp 47–56

Corticosteroid-Sparing Agents: New Treatment Options

Oren Tomkins-Netzer[a,b] · Simon R.J. Taylor[a,b,c] · Sue Lightman[a,b,c]

[a]Royal Surrey County Hospital, Guildford, and [b]Moorfields Eye Hospital and [c]UCL Institute of Ophthalmology, London, UK

Abstract

Corticosteroids form the cornerstone of treatment for noninfectious uveitis, but their safety profile and adverse effects render their use a double-edged sword. As a result, the local benefits of treating ocular inflammation may be outweighed by systemic adverse effects, and it is mainly for this reason that steroid-sparing agents are used. Most of these systemic immunomodulatory drugs used in ophthalmology have been adopted from other specialties, such as rheumatology and, while their safety profiles make them valid alternatives to long-term high-dose corticosteroids, systemic side effects still prove problematic for a significant proportion of patients. The desire to avoid these systemic side effects has driven the continuing search for effective agents with an improved safety profile, but also the increasing use of local drug administration, which avoids systemic side-effects, but may lead to ocular complications. Here we review both approaches and discuss the possible risks and benefits of each.

Corticosteroid therapy, though highly effective, is not without attendant side effects. It is associated with an increased risk of developing cataract or ocular hypertension, as well as of uncontrolled systemic glucose levels, systemic hypertension, Cushingoid effects, reduced bone mass and behavioural changes [1]. Indeed, the problems associated with using high-dose steroids over any period of time has led to the adoption of many second-line drugs with immunosuppressive properties in treating uveitis. Most of these were first used in the treatment of systemic autoimmune diseases, such as rheumatoid arthritis, or following organ transplantation. However, these compounds are also not without their own adverse reactions, and patients using these drugs are prone to diverse systemic adverse effects, depending on the specific compound, route of administration and underlying conditions. Commonly, these include disturbed liver function, increased susceptibility to infections, myelosuppression and, possibly, the late development of malignancies.

An alternative strategy to reduce these problems is to deliver drugs locally to the affected organ, i.e. the eye. Traditionally, the periocular route has been used, but more

Table 1. Corticosteroid-sparing drugs

Drug	Mode of action	Side effects
Methotrexate	Folic acid analogue	Stomatitis, bone marrow suppression, hepatotoxicity, nephrotoxicity
Azathioprine	Purine base analogue	Bone marrow suppression, hepatotoxicity
Mycophenolate mofetil	Selective purine synthesis inhibitor	Bone marrow suppression, hepatotoxicity
Cyclophosphamide	DNA alkylation	Haemorrhagic cystitis, bone marrow suppression, gastrointestinal toxicity, bladder and haematologic malignancies
Chlorambucil	DNA alkylation	Bone marrow suppression, gastrointestinal toxicity, haematologic malignancies
Cyclosporine	Calcineurin inhibitor	Hirsutism, gingival hyperplasia, nephrotoxicity, hypertension, hypercholesterolaemia, convulsions
Tacrolimus	Calcineurin inhibitor	ECG abnormalities, cardiomyopathy, chronic diarrhoea, lymphoproliferative disease, Infections
Infliximab	TNF-α antibody	Infusion reaction (fever, rash, dyspnoea, hypotension), headaches, anaphylaxis, susceptibility to tuberculosis, demyelinating disease
Adalimumab	Fully humanised TNF-α antibody	Headaches, rash, nausea, stomach upset, infections
Rituximab	Anti-CD20 antibody	Infusion reaction, systemic infections
IFN-α2a	Immunomodulatory cytokine	Flu-like symptoms, leucopoenia, central nervous system depression

recently, corticosteroids in the form of triamcinolone acetate have been injected into the vitreous cavity via an intravitreal injection. Further to this, long-acting implants have been developed. However, periocular and intraocular corticosteroids can cause the development of cataract or raised intraocular pressure, so newer agents have been tested to see if they can maintain similar efficacy with a reduced side effect profile.

Systemic Steroid-Sparing Agents

Systemic steroid-sparing agents can be divided into several main classes, each of which is associated with a different profile of efficacy and side effects (table 1).

Antimetabolites

These are a class of compounds that inhibit nucleic acid synthesis and cell proliferation, and are exemplified by methotrexate and azathioprine. Both of these drugs have been used for many years for immunosuppression in both organ transplantation and autoimmune diseases, and their relatively good safety profile and ease of use have made them a popular choice for many autoimmune conditions. Indeed, methotrexate has been successfully used in treating ocular inflammation for over 50 years, including juvenile idiopathic arthritis-associated uveitis [2], ocular sarcoidosis [3], scleritis [4] and refractory uveitis [5]. The Systemic Immunosupressive Therapy for Eyes (SITE) study is a recent, large survey of the use of steroid-sparing immunosuppressive agents in uveitis [6], and has provided valuable information about many of these immunosuppressive agents. In the study, 639 eyes were treated with methotrexate [7] and, at 12 months, 66% achieved corticosteroid-sparing control and 58% were able to reduce their steroid treatment to under 10 mg. Interestingly, however, the rate of onset of effect was slow, with many patients requiring a full 6 months of therapy before the full steroid-sparing effect was seen. 16% of patients in this study discontinued treatment due to side effects, the most common being gastrointestinal upset, bone marrow suppression or elevated liver enzymes.

Mycophenolate mofetil is a selective purine synthesis inhibitor which is also used to treat organ transplant rejection as well as autoimmune diseases. By inhibiting the de novo purine pathway, it selectively inhibits B and T lymphocytes, and is widely used at a dose of 500–1,500 mg twice a day [8–10]. Interestingly, it may achieve inflammation control faster than methotrexate or azathioprine [11], and it is also generally effective and well tolerated [12]. In the SITE study, 397 eyes were treated with mycophenolate mofetil [13] and complete control of inflammation for at least 28 days was achieved in 53% of patients at 6 months and 73% at 12 months. Similarly, systemic corticosteroid use was reduced to 10 mg/day or less in 41 and 55% of patients respectively. 20% of patients discontinued the drug, with the most frequent side effects being gastrointestinal disturbance and bone marrow suppression. Treatment is not recommended at doses over 3 g/day due to an increased risk of cytomegalovirus infection [14–16].

Alkylating Agents

The use of alkylating agents such as cyclophosphamide and chlorambucil is now restricted to a small number of causes of severe inflammatory disease as more effective and less toxic agents have become available. By alkylating DNA, they inhibit its synthesis and thus suppress the production of rapidly replicating cells. Cyclophosphamide is most commonly indicated for ocular involvement as part of systemic vasculitides such as granulomatosis with polyangiitis (Wegener's) [17], but can also be used in severe systemic lupus erythematosus. In the SITE study, it was shown to be effective in achieving inflammation control in over 75% of uveitis patients at 12 months [18]. Chlorambucil has been reported to be useful in treating Behçet's uveitis [19–21] and Vogt-Koyanagi-Harada syndrome [22], but concerns regarding its life-threatening side effects and toxicity have severely restricted its use [23]. Both agents are associated with myelosuppression and the development of malignancies.

T Cell Inhibitors

Uveitis is generally considered a T cell-mediated disease, and T cell inhibitors such as cyclosporin, tacrolimus and sirolimus have entered common usage as steroid-sparing agents. They affect the signal transduction of T lymphocytes, resulting in a reduction in T cell activity and hence leading to immunosuppression. Cyclosporin, initially introduced to preventing rejection in renal transplant patients, has also proven useful in treating ocular inflammation, and used to be the most commonly used second-line agent. In the SITE study, over 50% of patients that were treated with cyclosporin showed inflammation control at 12 months [24], and it has been found to be effective in treating severe posterior uveitis, such as Behçet's uveitis [25, 26], birdshot chorioretinopathy [27], serpiginous choroiditis [28] and sympathetic ophthalmia [29]. Cyclosporin can also be used topically to treat the inflammatory component of ocular surface disease such as severe dry eye [30, 31], but it is not effective in treating uveitis when administered in this form [32, 33]. Tacrolimus is similar, and its use has been reported in uveitis [34, 35], even in patients refractory to cyclosporine [36], but its side-effect profile is similar to that of cyclosporine, although the incidence of hypertension, hyperlipidaemia, hirsutism and gingival hyperplasia is said to be somewhat lower [37, 38].

Voclosporin is a new-generation calcineurin inhibitor that has recently entered clinical trials as an alternative to cyclosporin [39]. Unfortunately the results of the uveitis trials have been disappointing, with licensing proving difficult to obtain in both the US and Europe as a result. There is also little experience with sirolimus, but small case series have suggested it may be useful in some patients [40, 41].

Biologic Anti-Inflammatory Agents

Biologic agents are emerging as the most recent tools to inhibit systemic inflammation, and are a class of molecular agents that have specific targets within the immune system. The first biological agents to enter mainstream use in ophthalmology were the tumour necrosis factor-α (TNF-α) antagonists. These had previously been used in rheumatology and profoundly affect T cell-mediated inflammation. Infliximab and adalimumab are both monoclonal antibodies specific for TNF-α, but whereas infliximab is a chimeric molecule containing rodent antigens, adalimumab is fully humanised. Infliximab has been found to be effective in treating Behçet's uveitis patients, reducing the number of uveitis attacks compared with cyclosporine and other conventional agents [42–44]. There is less direct evidence for the use of adalimumab, but data from patients treated with adalimumab for ankylosing spondylitis have indicated that it can reduce the frequency of anterior uveitis flares in these patients by up to 50% [45, 46]. It is also given by subcutaneous injection rather than intravenous infusion, making it more convenient for the patient and cheaper to administer. Both drugs are associated with reactivation of latent tuberculosis infection and unmasking of multiple sclerosis (which is associated with intermediate uveitis), so careful pre-treatment screening is required [47, 48]. Additionally, infliximab may require additional immunosuppression to reduce the risk of developing antibodies to the murine fragment of the antibody, unlike the fully humanised adalimumab [49]. Etanercept is the third anti-TNF-α drug, but is a TNF-α receptor blocking protein. It has attained widespread use in treating rheumatological conditions, but is much less effective in uveitis [49, 50].

Rituximab is a biological agent that is forcing immunologists to rethink the basic pathophysiology of some immune-mediated diseases. This is a chimeric monoclonal antibody which leads to the depletion of peripheral B cells, but not plasma cells, by targeting the B cell-specific CD20 calcium channel [51]. It has been used successfully in a number of autoimmune diseases, and is licensed in the US for the treatment of rheumatoid arthritis [52–54], but its mechanism of action in T cell-mediated diseases is not yet entirely clear. There is, however, recent evidence that it may be useful in the treatment of scleritis and orbital disease secondary to granulomatosis with polyangiitis (Wegener's), as well as refractory uveitis [55–59]. Its safety profile is relatively good, and it is expected to overtake cyclophosphamide as the first-line choice for induction of remission in granulomatosis with polyangiitis (Wegener's).

Interferon (IFN)-α (2a and 2b) is an immunomodulatory cytokine which has also been studied in the treatment of refractory uveitis, and is thought to be capable of inducing disease remission through the activation of regulatory T cells, leading to the potential for its immunosuppressive effects to last long after the drug is discontinued [60]. Recent reports have suggested that patients with uveitis secondary to Behçet's disease that is refractory to conventional immunosuppression can respond to treatment with thrice-weekly administration of IFN-α [61, 62], with the patients in these studies suffering from fewer attacks and being able to reduce or stop their corticosteroid treatment. Interestingly, in one study 76% of patients remained in remission for an average of 12 months after treatment was stopped [63]. The most common side effects, reported in almost all patients, are flu-like symptoms, which may be quite debilitating; more severe side effects include leucopenia, thrombocytopenia and central nervous system effects (psychosis, depression) [64, 65]. IFN-α2a has also been reported to have some effect in treating serpiginous choroiditis [66], refractory cystoid macular oedema [67] and other causes of sight-threatening uveitis [68].

Other drugs which have been used in uveitis include daclizumab, which is a humanised monoclonal antibody directed at the IL-2 receptor. It was first used to improve the outcome of renal transplant patients and reduce the number of acute rejection episodes, but studies have suggested that it has some efficacy in treating intermediate and posterior uveitis. However, its side-effect profile is not good, and it is not in widespread use [69, 70]. Similarly, intravenous immunoglobulin has been reported to be effective in a few small case series [71].

Local Steroid-Sparing Agents

An alternative to reducing doses of systemic steroids by using systemic steroid-sparing agents is to switch treatment strategies and use local therapy, i.e. drug delivery via the periocular or intraocular routes [72–74]. However, although this reduces the risk of systemic side effects, the eye is placed at an increased risk of local side effects, such as cataract generation and raised intraocular pressure [73, 75–77]. These drugs typically also have a relatively short duration of effect, although, intravitreal steroid implants have been recently been developed that last for much longer, such as the Ozurdex (dexamethasone) and Retisert (fluocinolone) implants. Studies have shown they achieve good control of the inflammation, but are still related to an increased risk of ocular hypertension and cataract, particularly the long-lasting fluocinolone implant [78–81], which has driven the search for alternatives to steroid-based therapy.

One such alternative is intravitreal methotrexate, which has recently been reported in the treatment of uveitis and uveitis-related cystoid macular oedema [82]. In one small open-label study of fifteen eyes, up to two injections of 400 µg/0.1 ml methotrexate resulted in improvements in visual acuity and inflammatory indices. These improvements lasted for several months and relapses could be successfully treated with repeat injections. Recent animal models have also examined the safety of intravitreal sirolimus [83]. No toxicity was noted in histological sections, and clinical trials are now underway. Several studies have suggested intravitreal infliximab may be used to treat uveitis [84–87], but there is concern that it may generate severe intraocular inflammation, so such treatment is currently considered highly experimental [88].

Following on from their role in neovascular age-related macular degeneration and macular oedema secondary to diabetic maculopathy and retinal vein occlusion, anti-vascular endothelial growth factor drugs such as ranibizumab and bevacizumab have been used in uveitic cystoid macular oedema. Recent clinical studies have demonstrated that these drugs can reduce the central macular thickness and possibly improve visual acuity [89–91], but are significantly inferior to intravitreal steroids, unlike methotrexate, which seems to have a broadly comparable effect [82].

References

1 Sallam A, Taylor SR, Lightman S: Review and update of intraocular therapy in noninfectious uveitis. Curr Opin Ophthalmol 2011;22:517–522.

2 Foeldvari I, Wierk A: Methotrexate is an effective treatment for chronic uveitis associated with juvenile idiopathic arthritis. J Rheumatol 2005;32:362–365.

3 Dev S, McCallum RM, Jaffe GJ: Methotrexate treatment for sarcoid-associated panuveitis. Ophthalmology 1999;106:111–118.

4 Weinblatt ME, Coblyn JS, Fox DA, Fraser PA, et al: Efficacy of low-dose methotrexate in rheumatoid arthritis. N Engl J Med 1985;312:818–822.

5 Holz FG, Krastel H, Breitbart A, Schwarz-Eywill M, Pezzutto A, et al: Low-dose methotrexate treatment in noninfectious uveitis resistant to corticosteroids. Ger J Ophthalmol 1992;1:142–144.

6 Kempen JH, Daniel E, Gangaputra S, Dreger K, et al: Methods for identifying long-term adverse effects of treatment in patients with eye diseases: the Systemic Immunosuppressive Therapy for Eye Diseases (SITE) Cohort Study. Ophthalmic Epidemiol 2008;15:47–55.

7 Gangaputra S, Newcomb CW, Liesegang TL, et al: Methotrexate for ocular inflammatory diseases. Ophthalmology 2009;116:2188e1–2198e1.

8 Thorne JE, et al: Mycophenolate mofetil therapy for inflammatory eye disease. Ophthalmology 2005;112:1472–1477.

9 Teoh SC, et al: Mycophenolate mofetil for the treatment of uveitis. Am J Ophthalmol 2008;146:752–760, 760e1–e3.

10 Choudhary A, et al: Mycophenolate mofetil as an immunosuppressive agent in refractory inflammatory eye disease. J Ocul Pharmacol Ther 2006;22:168–175.

11 Galor A, et al: Comparison of antimetabolite drugs as corticosteroid-sparing therapy for noninfectious ocular inflammation. Ophthalmology 2008;115:1826–1832.

12 Doycheva D, et al: Long-term results of therapy with mycophenolate mofetil in chronic non-infectious uveitis. Graefes Arch Clin Exp Ophthalmol 2011;249:1235–1243.

13 Daniel E, et al: Mycophenolate mofetil for ocular inflammation. Am J Ophthalmol 2010;149:423–432, e1–e2.

14 European Mycophenolate Mofetil Cooperative Study Group: Placebo-controlled study of mycophenolate mofetil combined with cyclosporin and corticosteroids for prevention of acute rejection. Lancet 1995;345:1321–1325.

15 The Tricontinental Mycophenolate Mofetil Renal Transplantation Study Group: A blinded, randomized clinical trial of mycophenolate mofetil for the prevention of acute rejection in cadaveric renal transplantation. Transplantation 1996;61:1029–1037.

16 Sollinger HW: Mycophenolate mofetil for the prevention of acute rejection in primary cadaveric renal allograft recipients. U.S. Renal Transplant Mycophenolate Mofetil Study Group. Transplantation 1995;60:225–232.

17 Langford CA: Cyclophosphamide as induction therapy for Wegener's granulomatosis and microscopic polyangiitis. Clin Exp Immunol 2011;164(suppl 1):31–34.

18 Pujari SS, et al: Cyclophosphamide for ocular inflammatory diseases. Ophthalmology 2010;117:356–365.

19 Mudun BA, et al: Short-term chlorambucil for refractory uveitis in Behcet's disease. Ocul Immunol Inflamm 2001;9:219–229.

20 O'Duffy JD, Robertson DM, Goldstein NP: Chlorambucil in the treatment of uveitis and meningoencephalitis of Behcet's disease. Am J Med 1984;76:75–84.

21 Zakka FR, et al: Current trends in the management of ocular symptoms in Adamantiades-Behcet's disease. Clin Ophthalmol 2009;3:567–579.

22 Fang W, Yang P: Vogt-Koyanagi-Harada syndrome. Curr Eye Res 2008;33:517–523.

23 Goldstein DA, et al: Long-term follow-up of patients treated with short-term high-dose chlorambucil for sight-threatening ocular inflammation. Ophthalmology 2002;109:370–377.

24 Kacmaz RO, et al: Cyclosporine for ocular inflammatory diseases. Ophthalmology 2010;117:576–584.

25 Masuda K, et al: Double-masked trial of cyclosporin versus colchicine and long-term open study of cyclosporin in Behcet's disease. Lancet 1989;1:1093–1096.

26 Ben Ezra D, et al: Evaluation of conventional therapy versus cyclosporine A in Behcet's syndrome. Transplant Proc 1988;20(suppl 4):136–143.

27 Kiss S, et al: Long-term follow-up of patients with birdshot retinochoroidopathy treated with corticosteroid-sparing systemic immunomodulatory therapy. Ophthalmology 2005;112:1066–1071.

28 Araujo AA, et al: Early treatment with cyclosporin in serpiginous choroidopathy maintains remission and good visual outcome. Br J Ophthalmol 2000;84:979–982.

29 Vote BJ, et al: Changing trends in sympathetic ophthalmia. Clin Experiment Ophthalmol 2004;32: 542–545.
30 Malta JB, et al: Treatment of ocular graft-versus-host disease with topical cyclosporine 0.05%. Cornea 2010;29:1392–1396.
31 Roberts CW, Carniglia PE, Brazzo BG: Comparison of topical cyclosporine, punctal occlusion, and a combination for the treatment of dry eye. Cornea 2007;26:805–809.
32 Gumus K, et al: Topical cyclosporine A as a steroid-sparing agent in steroid-dependent idiopathic ocular myositis with scleritis: a case report and review of the literature. Eye Contact Lens 2009;35: 275–278.
33 Utine CA, Stern M, Akpek EK: Clinical review: topical ophthalmic use of cyclosporin A. Ocul Immunol Inflamm 2010;18:352–361.
34 Hogan AC, et al: Long-term efficacy and tolerance of tacrolimus for the treatment of uveitis. Ophthalmology 2007;114:1000–1006.
35 Figueroa MS, Ciancas E, Orte L: Long-term follow-up of tacrolimus treatment in immune posterior uveitis. Eur J Ophthalmol 2007;17:69–74.
36 Sloper CM, Powell RJ, Dua HS: Tacrolimus (FK506) in the treatment of posterior uveitis refractory to cyclosporine. Ophthalmology 1999;106:723–728.
37 Penninga L, et al: Tacrolimus versus cyclosporine as primary immunosuppression after heart transplantation: systematic review with meta-analyses and trial sequential analyses of randomised trials. Eur J Clin Pharmacol 2010;66:1177–1187.
38 Reyes J, et al: Long-term results after conversion from cyclosporine to tacrolimus in pediatric liver transplantation for acute and chronic rejection. Transplantation 2000;69:2573–2580.
39 Anglade E, Aspeslet LJ, Weiss SL: A new agent for the treatment of noninfectious uveitis: rationale and design of three LUMINATE (Lux Uveitis Multicenter Investigation of a New Approach to Treatment) trials of steroid-sparing voclosporin. Clin Ophthalmol 2008;2:693–702.
40 Shanmuganathan VA, et al: The efficacy of sirolimus in the treatment of patients with refractory uveitis. Br J Ophthalmol 2005;89:666–669.
41 Phillips BN, Wroblewski KJ: A retrospective review of oral low-dose sirolimus (rapamycin) for the treatment of active uveitis. J Ophthalmic Inflamm Infect 2011;1:29–34.
42 Tabbara KF, Ai-Hemidan AI: Infliximab effects compared to conventional therapy in the management of retinal vasculitis in Behcet disease. Am J Ophthalmol 2008;146:845e1–850e1.
43 Mushtaq B, et al: Adalimumab for sight-threatening uveitis in Behcet's disease. Eye (Lond) 2007;21: 824–825.
44 Taylor SR, et al: Behcet disease: visual prognosis and factors influencing the development of visual loss. Am J Ophthalmol 2011;152:1059–1066.
45 Guignard S, et al: Efficacy of tumour necrosis factor blockers in reducing uveitis flares in patients with spondylarthropathy: a retrospective study. Ann Rheum Dis 2006;65:1631–1634.
46 Rudwaleit M, et al: Effectiveness, safety, and predictors of good clinical response in 1250 patients treated with adalimumab for active ankylosing spondylitis. J Rheumatol 2009;36:801–808.
47 Kim EM, et al: Incidence of tuberculosis among Korean patients with ankylosing spondylitis who are taking tumor necrosis factor blockers. J Rheumatol 2011;38:2218–2223.
48 Lamprecht P: TNF-alpha inhibitors in systemic vasculitides and connective tissue diseases. Autoimmun Rev 2005;4:28–34.
49 Jap A, Chee SP: Immunosuppressive therapy for ocular diseases. Curr Opin Ophthalmol 2008;19: 535–540.
50 Tak PP, Kalden JR: Advances in rheumatology: new targeted therapeutics. Arthritis Res Ther 2011; 13(suppl 1):S5.
51 Stashenko P, et al: Characterization of a human B lymphocyte-specific antigen. J Immunol 1980;125: 1678–1685.
52 Bar-Or A, et al: Rituximab in relapsing-remitting multiple sclerosis: a 72-week, open-label, phase I trial. Ann Neurol 2008;63:395–400.
53 Leandro MJ, et al: B-cell depletion in the treatment of patients with systemic lupus erythematosus: a longitudinal analysis of 24 patients. Rheumatology (Oxford) 2005;44:1542–1545.
54 Mease PJ, et al: Improved health-related quality of life for patients with active rheumatoid arthritis receiving rituximab: Results of the Dose-Ranging Assessment: International Clinical Evaluation of Rituximab in Rheumatoid Arthritis (DANCER) Trial. J Rheumatol 2008;35:20–30.
55 Taylor SR, et al: Rituximab is effective in the treatment of refractory ophthalmic Wegener's granulomatosis. Arthritis Rheum 2009;60:1540–1547.
56 Tappeiner C, et al: Rituximab as a treatment option for refractory endogenous anterior uveitis. Ophthalmic Res 2007;39:184–186.
57 Cheung CM, Murray PI, Savage CO: Successful treatment of Wegener's granulomatosis associated scleritis with rituximab. Br J Ophthalmol 2005;89: 1542.

58 Davatchi F, et al: Rituximab in intractable ocular lesions of Behcet's disease; randomized single-blind control study (pilot study). Int J Rheum Dis 2010; 13:246–252.
59 Sadreddini S, et al: Treatment of retinal vasculitis in Behcet's disease with rituximab. Mod Rheumatol 2008;18:306–308.
60 de Smet MD, et al: Understanding uveitis: the impact of research on visual outcomes. Prog Retin Eye Res 2011;30:452–470.
61 Sobaci G, et al: Safety and effectiveness of interferon alpha-2a in treatment of patients with Behcet's uveitis refractory to conventional treatments. Ophthalmology 2010;117:1430–1435.
62 Kötte I, et al: The use of interferon alpha in Behçet disease: review of the literature. Semin Arthritis Rheum 2004;33:320–335.
63 Onal S, et al: Long-term efficacy and safety of low-dose and dose-escalating interferon alfa-2a therapy in refractory Behcet uveitis. Arch Ophthalmol 2011;129:288–294.
64 Krause L, et al: Longterm visual prognosis of patients with ocular Adamantiades-Behcet's disease treated with interferon-alpha-2a. J Rheumatol 2008; 35:896–903.
65 Gueudry J, et al: Long-term efficacy and safety of low-dose interferon alpha2a therapy in severe uveitis associated with Behcet disease. Am J Ophthalmol 2008;146:837e1–844e1.
66 Sobaci G, Bayraktar Z, Bayer A: Interferon alpha-2a treatment for serpiginous choroiditis. Ocul Immunol Inflamm 2005;13:59–66.
67 Deuter CM, et al: Interferon alfa-2a: a new treatment option for long lasting refractory cystoid macular edema in uveitis? A pilot study. Retina 2006;26: 786–791.
68 Bodaghi B, et al: Efficacy of interferon alpha in the treatment of refractory and sight threatening uveitis: a retrospective monocentric study of 45 patients. Br J Ophthalmol 2007;91:335–339.
69 Sen HN, et al: High-dose daclizumab for the treatment of juvenile idiopathic arthritis-associated active anterior uveitis. Am J Ophthalmol 2009;148: 696e1–703e1.
70 Wroblewski K, et al: Long-term daclizumab therapy for the treatment of noninfectious ocular inflammatory disease. Can J Ophthalmol 2011;46:322–328.
71 Onal S, Foster CS, Ahmed AR: Efficacy of intravenous immunoglobulin treatment in refractory uveitis. Ocul Immunol Inflamm 2006;14:367–374.
72 Androudi S, et al: Safety and efficacy of intravitreal triamcinolone acetonide for uveitic macular edema. Ocul Immunol Inflamm 2005;13:205–212.
73 Kok H, et al: Outcome of intravitreal triamcinolone in uveitis. Ophthalmology 2005;112:1916e1–1917e1.
74 Young S, et al: Safety and efficacy of intravitreal triamcinolone for cystoid macular oedema in uveitis. Clin Experiment Ophthalmol 2001;29:2–6.
75 Jonas JB, et al: Intraocular pressure elevation after intravitreal triamcinolone acetonide injection. Ophthalmology 2005;112:593–598.
76 Roth DB, et al: Long-term incidence and timing of intraocular hypertension after intravitreal triamcinolone acetonide injection. Ophthalmology 2009; 116:455–460.
77 Smithen LM, et al: Intravitreal triamcinolone acetonide and intraocular pressure. Am J Ophthalmol 2004;138:740–743.
78 Haller JA, et al: Dexamethasone intravitreal implant in patients with macular edema related to branch or central retinal vein occlusion twelve-month study results. Ophthalmology 2011;118:2453–2460.
79 Jaffe GJ, et al: Fluocinolone acetonide implant (Retisert) for noninfectious posterior uveitis: thirty-four-week results of a multicenter randomized clinical study. Ophthalmology 2006;113:1020–1027.
80 Kempen JH, et al: Randomized comparison of systemic anti-inflammatory therapy versus fluocinolone acetonide implant for intermediate, posterior, and panuveitis: The Multicenter Uveitis Steroid Treatment Trial. Ophthalmology 2011;118: 1916–1926.
81 Lowder C, et al: Dexamethasone intravitreal implant for noninfectious intermediate or posterior uveitis. Arch Ophthalmol 2011;129:545–553.
82 Taylor SR, et al: Intraocular methotrexate in the treatment of uveitis and uveitic cystoid macular edema. Ophthalmology 2009;116:797–801.
83 Douglas LC, et al: Ocular toxicity and distribution of subconjunctival and intravitreal rapamycin in horses. J Vet Pharmacol Ther 2008;31:511–516.
84 Farvardin M, et al: Intravitreal infliximab for the treatment of sight-threatening chronic noninfectious uveitis. Retina 2010;30:1530–1535.
85 Theodossiadis PG, et al: Intravitreal administration of the anti-TNF monoclonal antibody infliximab in the rabbit. Graefes Arch Clin Exp Ophthalmol 2009; 247:273–281.
86 Giansanti F, et al: Ocular safety of infliximab in rabbit and cell culture models. J Ocul Pharmacol Ther 2010;26:65–71.
87 Hosseini H, et al: Intravitreal infliximab in experimental endotoxin-induced uveitis. Eur J Ophthalmol 2009;19:818–823.

88 Pulido JS, et al: More questions than answers: a call for a moratorium on the use of intravitreal infliximab outside of a well-designed trial. Retina 2010; 30:1–5.
89 Weiss K, et al: Intravitreal VEGF levels in uveitis patients and treatment of uveitic macular oedema with intravitreal bevacizumab. Eye (Lond) 2009;23: 1812–1818.
90 Mackensen F, et al: Intravitreal bevacizumab (avastin) as a treatment for refractory macular edema in patients with uveitis: a pilot study. Retina 2008;28: 41–45.
91 Acharya NR, Hong KC, Lee SM: Ranibizumab for refractory uveitis-related macular edema. Am J Ophthalmol 2009;148:303e2–309e2.

Prof. Sue Lightman
UCL Institute of Ophthalmology
Moorfields Eye Hospital, 162 City Road
London EC1V 2PD (UK)
Tel. +44 207 566 2266, E-Mail s.lightman@ucl.ac.uk

Miserocchi E, Modorati G, Foster CS (eds): New Treatments in Noninfectious Uveitis.
Dev Ophthalmol. Basel, Karger, 2012, vol 51, pp 57–62

Mycophenolate Mofetil Use in the Treatment of Noninfectious Uveitis

Dino D. Klisovic

Midwest Retina, Dublin, Ohio, USA

Abstract

Mycophenolate mophetil (MMP) is a potent immunomodulatory drug that inhibits the function of T and B lymphocytes. It is used successfully in the treatment of recurrent noninfectious uveitis in adults and children. MMF can be used alone or in combination with other immunomodulatory drugs (biologics or calcineurin inhibitors) for moderate and severe cases of anterior, intermediate and posterior uveitis. It can also be used for treatment of patients with scleritis and ocular cicatricial pemphigoid.

Mycophenolate mofetil (MMF; CellCept, Roche) is a 2-morpholinoethyl ester of mycophenolic acid (MPA). MMF is quickly transformed into an active drug, MPA – an uncompetitive and reversible inhibitor of inosine monophosphate dehydrogenase (IMPDH) [1, 2]. IMPDH is crucial in de novo synthesis of guanosine monophosphate, which in turn is essential in RNA and DNA synthesis in rapidly proliferating cells such as activated T and B lymphocytes. Unlike the rest of the cells in the human body, T and B lymphocytes are unable to use the salvage pathway of purine nucleotide synthesis which bypasses the IMPDH step. In addition, MPA is a fivefold more potent inhibitor of the type II isoform of IMPDH that is expressed in activated T and B lymphocytes than of the housekeeping type I isoform that is expressed in most cell types. Dependence of lymphocytes on de novo synthesis of guanosine monophosphate and the expression of type II IMPDH isoform explains the preferential effect of MPA on activated lymphocytes [1]. The effect of MMF on lymphocyte function is complex and involves: suppression of the proliferation of cytotoxic T cells, inhibition of adhesion and penetration of CD4+ and CD8+ T cells, inhibition of recruitment of monocytes, inhibition of proliferation of B lymphocytes, decrease in production of antibodies and decrease in production of proinflammatory cytokines [1].

MMF has been most widely used to suppress allograft rejection of solid organs (e.g. kidney and heart). Its excellent immunomodulatory properties were recognized by uveitis specialists, and over the last decade MMF became an important tool in the armamentarium of uveitis specialists worldwide. MMF can be used alone or in combination with other steroid-sparing immunomodulatory drugs (IMDs) in treatment of both adults and children with all types of uveitis including anterior, intermediate and posterior uveitis cases. It is also valuable in the treatment of scleritis, ocular cicatricial pemphigoid and orbital inflammatory pseudotumor.

Effectiveness of MMF in the treatment of noninfectious uveitis was first described in 1999 [3]. MMF was used in 11 patients with severe uveitis and scleritis that were failing combinations of prednisone and azathioprine (AZA) or prednisone and cyclosporine (CSA). MMF was used instead of AZA with prednisone or was added to a combination of prednisone and CSA. Addition of MMF allowed reduction of prednisone dose and led to improvement in inflammation in 10 out of 11 patients.

Similar results were obtained in two larger studies that evaluated MMF in the treatment of patients with steroid-dependent or steroid-resistant uveitis [4, 5]. Those studies included patients that were affected by uveitis, scleritis, ocular cicatricial pemphigoid and orbital inflammatory pseudotumor. MMF was used as a monotherapy or as an addition to another IMD. Control of intraocular inflammation was achieved in 65% of patients treated with MMF as monotherapy. Steroid-sparing effect was achieved in 54% of patients. The median time to treatment success was 3.5 months with the majority of treatment successes occurring within the first 6 months of treatment. Of the patients who had steroid-sparing success, 70% were able to taper to less than 5 mg of prednisone daily and 40% were able to stop prednisone without relapse of inflammation. MMF was effective as a steroid-sparing drug regardless of the type of intraocular inflammation.

A study from the UK investigated steroid-sparing effects of MMF treatment (alone or in combination with other IMDs) in 100 patients with uveitis. It revealed 85% probability of tapering prednisone dose to less than 10 mg/day after one year of MMF treatment [6].

The largest study done so far encompassed 236 patients with uveitis, scleritis and OCP that were treated at four subspecialty clinics from 1995 to 2007 [7]. Patients were treated with MMF and various doses of prednisone. By 12 months of treatment, 44% of patients achieved complete control of inflammation with less than 5 mg of prednisone daily and 55% of patients achieved the same control with less than 10 mg daily. In addition, proportion of complete inflammation control at 1 year was 73% overall and ranged from 71% for panuveitis to 86% for scleritis.

Sobrin et al. [8] specifically analyzed the effect of MMF on uveitis and scleritis control in 85 patients who failed or were intolerant of previous methotrexate (MTX) treatment. Fifty-five percent of those patients had adequate control with MMF alone. Patients with scleritis and juvenile idiopathic arthritis-associated uveitis responded less favorably to MMF monotreatment compared to patients with other types of ocular inflammation. Seventy-three percent of patients who concomitantly used prednisone were able to lower the prednisone dose to less than 10 mg a day.

A study done by Galor et al. [9] provided a direct comparison of efficacy and side effects of the three most commonly used IMDs – MTX, AZA and MMF in a group of 257 patients that had active uveitis (anterior, intermediate or posterior) or scleritis. Patients were treated with one of three IMDs as a first line of treatment. MMF achieved treatment success more rapidly than MTX or AZA. The median time to treatment success, in months, was 4.0 for MMF, 4.8 for AZA and 6.5 for MTX. In addition, the proportion of patients with treatment success after 6 months of treatment was highest in the MMF group – 70 vs. 42% for MTX and 58% for AZA. Of those drugs, AZA had the highest rate of side effects compared to the other two drugs – gastrointestinal upset, hematological abnormalities and liver dysfunction.

Mycophenolate Mofetil in the Treatment of Pediatric Uveitis

Diagnosis and treatment of all forms of uveitis in children are associated with numerous difficulties such as delay in diagnosis, difficulties in examining children, and early development of cataract that can lead to amblyopia. In addition, some forms of uveitis, such as pars planitis can have a more aggressive course in children than adults. If not treated early and very aggressively, uveitis can have more devastating consequences on vision in children than in adults. Therefore, there is great need to bring intraocular inflammation under complete control very quickly. This task can be difficult to achieve if (a) an inflammation responds poorly to the first IMD used or (b) if a relapse occurs despite initial inflammation control that cannot be brought under control with further increase in IMD dose. The latter problem can be unrelated to other medical problems or, more commonly, it can be seen in winter months after a bout of cold/flu or if the IMD had to be stopped for a short time in order to treat bacterial infection or to perform immunization. This problem can be seen relatively often with MTX treatment, which is frequently used as a first IMD in children (especially for JRA-associated uveitis). Unfortunately, MTX has a failure rate of approximately 35–40% in all uveitis cases.

Two recent papers described the efficacy of MMF in the treatment of children with anterior, intermediate and posterior uveitis who have previously failed other steroid-sparing IMDs such as MTX, CSA and biologics such as adalimumab, infliximab or etanercept [10, 11]. Chang et al. [11] followed 52 patients over a period of 4 years, and showed that 73% of those patients achieved inflammation control following 2 months of MMF monotherapy. Of those patients, 66% achieved durable disease control (quiescence for at least 2 years on MMF monotherapy and no more than 2 flare-ups that were treated with increase in MMF dose) and 33% achieved short-term inflammation control (quiescence less than 2 years, no more than one flare-up treated with an increase in MMF dose). Visual acuity worsened in 6% of patients and remained stable or improved in 94% of patients. A minority of patients (12%) had to discontinue MMF due to side effects – most commonly gastrointestinal upset. The dose of MMF utilized in children is 600 mg/m^2 twice daily.

All studies mentioned so far in this paper have several major limitations: (a) retrospective review; (b) lack of proper randomization; (c) performed at tertiary academic centers, so there is an inherent bias toward patients with more severe inflammation that failed treatment(s) with other IMDs. However, in spite of all shortcomings, results of those studies are very encouraging to all of us who deal on a daily basis with patients who struggle with chronic uveitis.

Treatment Algorithm(s) in the Use of Mycophenolate Mofetil in Uveitis Patients

The choice of IMD in the treatment of any patient with uveitis depends on a variety of factors including: the type and severity of inflammation, amount of intraocular damage, presence or absence of systemic comorbidities, previous failure of other IMDs or contraindications for their use. With these factors in mind, a treatment algorithm for the use of MMF in uveitis patients will be described.

MMF is typically employed as a second-line IMD in the treatment of mild to moderate cases of anterior uveitis (i.e. HLA-B27 anterior uveitis, JRA, etc.) and scleritis. Namely, if not contraindicated, those patients are first treated with MTX or AZT. If those two drugs are not able to control inflammation (40% failure rate with MTX) or their use is limited by side effects (i.e. fatigue, leukocytopenia), MTX or AZT are stopped and MMF is started. MMF, like MTX or AZT, takes approximately 6 weeks to show clinical effect. Treatment is initiated at 500 mg twice a day. Provided that the patient tolerates the drug well, the dose is increased to 1,000 mg twice a day (starting dose for an adult) and continued for 5–6 weeks. Depending on the degree to which the inflammation is controlled, the dose of MMF can be increased by 500 mg every 6 weeks if necessary until the maximum daily dose is achieved – 1,500 mg twice a day. We do not believe in using the small dose of MMF (e.g. 2,000 mg a day) and adding steroids (orally, intra- or periocular injections) to control inflammation. If inflammation is not optimally controlled on maximum-dose MMF, addition of a second IMF such as CSA or a biological drug such as infliximab is indicated.

Complete blood count and liver function tests are checked every 6 weeks. Effort should be made to keep WBC above 4,000–4,500 cells/µl, neutrophil count above 1,500 cells/µl and platelets above 75,000 cells/µl. If the WBC drops below 4,000 cells/µl while on MMF treatment, the MMF should be temporarily discontinued and the WBC rechecked on a weekly basis. Once the WBC is above 4,000 cells/µl, MMF should be restarted, but at a half-dose. Patients that have active chronic uveitis and low WBC (~4,000 cells/µl) before the start of immunomodulatory therapy often represent a particular problem for the treating uveitis specialist. In those patients, MMF may be initiated at a low dose – 500 mg once a day along with CSA (1–3 mg/kg/day)

Table 1. Diagnoses that may warrant MMF as a first line of treatment

Moderate or severe bilateral posterior uveitis
Inflammation in monocular patients
Birdshot retinochoroidopathy
Vogt-Koyanaga-Harada disease
Retinal vasculitis with optic nerve involvement
Behçet's disease
Sympathetic ophthalmia
Orbital inflammatory pseudotumor
Ocular cicatricial pemphigoid

and a small dose of prednisone (2.5–5.0 mg/day), which often keeps WBC from getting too low. The dose of MMF in those patients is slowly increased until the therapeutic effect is achieved provided that WBC stays above 3,500 cells/μl.

MMF is an excellent first-line treatment in patients who have recently been diagnosed with severe bilateral posterior uveitis and in monocular patients with moderate to severe inflammation. Table 1 lists diagnoses that may warrant MMF as a first line of treatment.

In patients with above-listed diagnoses, a combination of MMF (up to 3,000 mg a day) and CSA (up to 3 mg/kg/day) may be more effective, especially in patients with BSRC. In addition, when it is imperative that a severe intraocular inflammation has to be put under control very quickly (i.e. Behçet's disease), concomitant initiation of oral prednisone (1 mg/kg/day) or intravenous methylprednisolone (1–2 g/day), along with MMF (1,000 mg b.i.d.) and CSA (1–3 mg/day divided in two doses) should be used. As the inflammation is controlled, prednisone is slowly tapered after 6 weeks, and doses of MMF and CSA are adjusted based on complete blood count and the amount of inflammation. If the inflammation is well controlled during the first 6–9 months of treatment, CSA can often be discontinued and MMF can be continued as monotherapy.

Sometimes, in order to achieve complete cessation of intraocular inflammation, a combination of maximum dose MMF and CSA can be supplemented with: (a) biological drugs such as adalimumab (Humira) or infliximab (Remicade) or (b) weekly MTX (less preferred, but helpful combination in some difficult cases or in cases where expensive biological drugs cannot be used).

The goal of immunomodulatory therapy in chronic uveitis patients is a durable (at least 2 years) control of intraocular inflammation using steroid-sparing IMDs (alone or in combination) without concomitant use of oral or topical steroids. After 2 years of quiescence, a slow taper of IMD is done within no less than 6 months. In patients whose inflammation does not reactivate during the taper period, one can expect a 70–90% long-term remission rate, which is often equivalent to cure in those patients. Complete quiescence of inflammation for 2 years cannot be easily and quickly achieved in many patients. The road to durable remission is often long and frustrating and requires a strong commitment from both the patient and the treating uveitis specialist. MMF has become an invaluable asset in this noble and important quest.

References

1. Allison AC: Mechanism of action of mycophenolate mofetil. Lupus 2005;14:2–8.
2. Tett SE, Saint-Marcoux F, Staaz CE, Brunet M, Vinks AA, Miura M, Marquet P, Kuypers DR, von Gelder T, Cattaneo D: Mycophenolate, clinical pharmacokinetics, formulations and methods for assessing drug exposure. Transplant Rev 2011;25:47–57.
3. Larkin G, Lightman S: Mycophenolate mofetil. A useful immunosuppressive in inflammatory eye disease. Ophthalmology 1999;106:370–374.
4. Baltatzis S, Tufail F, Yu EN, Vredevled CM, Foster CS: Mycophenolate mofetil as an immunomodulatory agent in the treatment of chronic ocular inflammatory disorders. Ophthalmology 2003;110:1061–1065.
5. Thorne JE, Jabs DA, Qazi FA, Nguyen QD, Kempen JH, Dunn JP: Mycophenolate mofetil therapy for inflammatory eye disease. Ophthalmology 2005;112:1472–1477.
6. Teoh SC, Hogan AC, Dick AD, Lee RW: Mycophenolate mofetil for the treatment of uveitis. Am J Ophthalmol 2008;146:752–760.
7. Daniel E, Thorne JE, Newcomb CW, Pujari SS, Kaçmaz RO, Levy-Clarke GA, Nussenblatt RB, Rosenbaum JT, Suhler EB, Foster CS, Jabs D, Kempen JH: Mycophenolate mofetil for ocular inflammation. Am J Ophthalmol 2010;149:423–432.
8. Sobrin L, Christen E, Foster CS: Mycophenolate mofetil after methotrexate failure or intolerance in the treatment of scleritis and uveitis. Ophthalmology 2008;115:1416–1421.
9. Galor A, Jabs DA, Leder HA, Kedhar SR, Dunn JP, Peters GB 3rd, Thorne JE: Comparison of antimetabolite drugs as corticosteroid-sparing therapy for noninfectious ocular inflammation. Ophthalmology 2008;115;1826–1832.
10. Doycheva D, Deuter C, Stuebinger N, Biester S, Zierhut M: Mycophenolate mofetil in the treatment of uveitis in children. Br J Ophthalmol 2007;91:180–184.
11. Chang PY, Giuliari GP, Shaikh M, Thakuria P, Makhoul D, Foster CS: Mycophenolate mofetil monotherapy in the management of paediatric uveitis. Eye 2011;25:427–435.

Dino D. Klisovic, MD
Midwest Retina
6655 Post Road
Dublin, OH 43016 (USA)
Tel. +1 614 339 8500, E-Mail dklisov@yahoo.com

Miserocchi E, Modorati G, Foster CS (eds): New Treatments in Noninfectious Uveitis.
Dev Ophthalmol. Basel, Karger, 2012, vol 51, pp 63–78

Anti-Tumor Necrosis Factor-α Agents in Noninfectious Uveitis

Julie Gueudry[a] · Phuc LeHoang[b] · Bahram Bodaghi[b]

[a]Department of Ophthalmology, Charles Nicolle University Hospital, Rouen, and
[b]Department of Ophthalmology, University of Paris VI, Pitié-Salpêtrière Hospital, Paris, France

Abstract

Anti-tumor necrosis factor-α (anti-TNF-α) agents represent a major breakthrough for the therapeutic management of different autoimmune conditions. Noninfectious uveitis may lead to various sight-threatening complications. Hence, from extrapolation of the benefit observed in autoimmune systemic diseases, anti-TNF-α agents are widely used in the treatment of noninfectious uveitis. However, their use remains mostly 'off-label' in this indication, and the lack of evidence from randomized controlled studies limits a rationale choice. This review gives an update on the management of uveitis with TNF-α inhibitors, highlighting important issues, including initiation time, type of molecule, duration of therapy but also major adverse events.

Over the past 2 decades, therapy for a number of inflammatory diseases has developed into a highly differentiated approach with an increasing number of drug options. The introduction of anti-tumor necrosis factor-α (TNF-α) agents has revolutionized the treatment of rheumatic diseases such as rheumatoid arthritis, spondyloarthropathies and idiopathic juvenile arthritis as well as inflammatory bowel disease. Hence, anti-TNF-α agents have become a valuable addition to the therapeutic armamentarium for patients with refractory uveitis or intolerant to conventional treatment. However, due to the lack of evidence from randomized controlled trials, their use in uveitis remains 'off-label' in most countries. The purpose of this review is to stress current evidence on the use of these drugs, highlighting various possible choices of molecules and treatment strategies in intraocular inflammatory diseases.

Tumor Necrosis Factor-α

TNF-α is a highly potent proinflammatory cytokine with a wide range of activities in both inflammatory and immune responses. First characterized in 1985 [1], TNF-α is synthesized by T helper cells and by activated macrophages, monocytes, neutrophils, and endothelial cells. It is primarily produced as a membrane-bound surface molecule, and a soluble form is created by proteolytic cleavage from the cell surface. It activates other cytokines, upregulates endothelial adhesion molecules, increases cell-mediated immunity and enhances granuloma formation and maintenance [2]. Therefore, TNF-α plays an important role in host defense against infectious agents. Particularly, data have suggested that TNF-mediated formation and maintenance of granuloma is fundamental for controlling *Mycobacterium tuberculosis* infection [3]. TNF-α achieves all its different cellular and pathological effects by its binding to either the TNFR1 (or p55) or TNFR2 (or p75) receptor subtype. TNF-α receptors on cells are stimulated by both soluble and transmembrane forms of TNF-α. However, soluble TNF-α mainly stimulates TNFR1 and membrane TNF-α mainly stimulates TNFR2 [2].

TNF-α is involved in the pathogenesis of many inflammatory disorders including noninfectious uveitis. Evidence for its pivotal role comes from experimental studies. A high TNF-α level was identified in the uvea and retina [4], in the aqueous humor and serum [5] of rats with endotoxin-induced uveitis. An intraocular high TNF-α level was identified in rats with experimental autoimmune uveitis [6, 7]. Moreover, intravitreal TNF-α injection in rabbits [8] and rats [9] was able to induce acute uveitis. There is evidence of raised TNF-α levels in ocular fluids of patients with uveitis [10, 11]. Interestingly, in endotoxin-induced uveitis, paradoxical effects of TNF blockage were also reported [12, 13].

Anti-TNF-α Agents

There are currently five anti-TNF-α agents available (table 1).

Etanercept

Etanercept is a fusion protein combining two human p75 TNF-α receptors. While both infliximab and adalimumab bind effectively to the soluble and transmembrane forms of TNF-α, etanercept forms less stable bonds with TNF-α, particularly the transmembrane form [14]. Etanercept does not appear to be an effective treatment for uveitis. Randomized controlled trials comparing etanercept with placebo in the treatment of chronic noninfectious uveitis [15], uveitis associated with juvenile idiopathic arthritis [16], and uveitis associated with sarcoidosis [17] found no benefit over placebo. Finally, retrospective studies showed that etanercept seems to be less efficacious than infliximab [18–20], as in a recent meta-analysis [21] of data from 4 placebo-controlled studies with anti-TNF agents in ankylosing spondylitis.

Table 1. Comparison of different anti-TNF-α agents

Agents	Etanercept	Infliximab	Adalimumab	Certolizumab pegol	Golimumab
Year approved for use in the US	1998	1999	2002	2008	2009
Indications					
Rheumatoid arthritis	×	×	×	×[a]	×
JIA	×		×		
Ankylosing spondylitis	×	×	×		×
Psoriatic arthritis	×	×	×		×
Plaque psoriasis	×	×	×		
Crohn's disease					
Adult		×	×	×	
Pediatric		×			
Ulcerative colitis		×			
Route of administration	s.c.	i.v.	s.c.	s.c.	s.c.
Maintenance dosing interval	1 week[b]	6–8 weeks[c]	2 weeks	1 month	1 month

[a] In 2009, approved for use only in the treatment of rheumatoid arthritis in Europe.
[b] May be given twice weekly.
[c] The routine dosing interval is 6 weeks in patients with ankylosing spondylitis.

Infliximab

Infliximab is a murine-human chimeric antibody against TNF-α. It binds soluble and transmembrane forms of TNF-α with high affinity. The usual loading dose is 3–5 mg/kg body weight, intravenously, which can be increased to 10 mg/kg. Infusions are repeated after 2 and 6 weeks and, depending on clinical scores, every 4–8 weeks. Several studies reviewed infliximab efficacy in preventing uveitis relapses, in maintaining visual acuity and in the ability to taper corticosteroids and immunosuppressive agents [22, 23].

Adalimumab

Adalimumab is a fully humanized monoclonal antibody against TNF-α. It also binds to the soluble and transmembrane forms of TNF-α. Adalimumab has the technical advantage of a subcutaneous administration and is injected at a dosage of 40 mg every 2 weeks in adults. Since 2006, adalimumab has been used with positive results in refractory uveitis, and many types of uveitis seem to respond to adalimumab [24]. Moreover, the first prospective comparative study, however without randomization, between infliximab and adalimumab in childhood chronic uveitis suggests the potential superiority of adalimumab [25].

New TNF-α Blockers

Golimumab is a fully humanized anti-TNF-α monoclonal antibody, which is delivered monthly by the subcutaneous route. It binds to both soluble and transmembrane forms of human TNF-α. The constant regions of the heavy and light chains of golimumab are identical to those of infliximab in terms of the amino acid sequence. The variable region is specific for human TNF-α. It was approved in the United States in 2009 for use with methotrexate in adults with moderate to severe active rheumatoid arthritis and with or without methotrexate in adults with active psoriatic arthritis or active ankylosing spondylitis. In 2011, the two first cases of uveitis treated with golimumab were reported with encouraging results [26]. Certolizumab-pegol is a humanized PEGylated anti-TNF-α antibody. The pegylation of the antibody delays the elimination and thus provides a longer half-life. Certolizumab is the only TNF-α inhibitor that uses PEGylated technology. At the time of writing this chapter (December 2011), there is no scientific report on the use of certolizumab pegol in uveitis.

Anti-TNF-α Agents: Treatment Indications for Use

Behçet's Disease-Associated Uveitis

Behçet's disease (BD) is a chronic, relapsing, inflammatory disorder. Uveitis is one of the most severe complications of the disease. Visual prognosis has improved in recent years with the increasing use of immunosuppressive agents. Nevertheless, in a few cases, uveitis remains refractory to conventional therapy; and despite these aggressive strategies, blindness may occur. Recent results based on the use of anti-TNF agents highlight their significant efficacy [27]. Concerning the use of anti-TNF-α agents in BD, there is only one randomized, double-blind, placebo-control trial that evaluated the effect of etanercept on mucocutaneous manifestations and arthritis. Etanercept was beneficial for most of these manifestations, but no data about ocular involvement were available in that study [28]. Administration of infliximab for ocular inflammation in BD was first reported in 2001 [29]. The published evidence consists mainly of reports of the open use of infliximab, recently reviewed. Among these 158 reported patients, a rapid and dramatic improvement of visual acuity and decrease in ocular inflammation starting

24 h after infliximab was almost always reported [30]. A significant reduction in subsequent attacks of uveitis was achieved in 89% of these patients (65% was reported as complete). As BD is one of the most serious and sight-threatening clinical uveitis entities, infliximab was approved in Japan for the treatment of 'Behcet's disease complicated with refractory uveoretinitis, which does not respond to conventional therapies' (Osaka, Japan, January 26, 2007, JCN Newswire) despite the lack of randomized controlled trials available. Moreover, the EULAR recommendations [31] on the treatment of BD were published including anti-TNF-α use. Infliximab dose of 10 mg/kg might not be superior to 5 mg/kg in efficacy and repeated infusions are needed [32]. The recommendations on the use of anti-TNF-α agents in BD by an expert panel explained that in acute, unilateral, posterior uveitis with significant reduction in visual acuity (<20/100), as well as in cases with inflammation at the level of the macular area and those with bilateral involvement, infliximab could be used as a first-line agent to achieve a fast-onset response. In patients with two or more relapses/year despite, or intolerant to, adequate doses of azathioprine and/or cyclosporin A, or, interferon (IFN)-α2a, combined with prednisolone (<7.5 mg/day), infliximab can be used as a maintenance regimen [27]. However, it is important to note that there are no data supporting continuous use of infliximab as a monotherapy [27]. Even though IFN-α2a seems to be an alternative to anti-TNF-α drugs [33], anti-TNF-α seems to be appropriate, particularly in case of IFN-α2a failure [27, 29, 34, 35]. Use of anti-TNF-α agents in BD was principally evaluated as an add-on therapy. Actually, at initiation of treatment with infliximab, concomitant administration of immunosuppressive agents was discontinued in some studies, whereas corticosteroid therapy was not [30]. Nonetheless, a prospective comparative study comparing different treatment approaches for acute panuveitis attacks in BD have been recently reported [36]. It shows that infliximab (5 mg/kg), when given at the onset of an acute panuveitis attack, exerts a significantly faster and more effective effect in suppressing ocular inflammation than intravitreal triamcinolone (4 mg) or high-dose methylprednisolone (3-day course, 1 g/day). Given that control of acute ocular inflammation in BD is mandatory to avoid permanent visual loss, an intravenous infliximab infusion should be always considered for panuveitis attacks in BD. Few reports on adalimumab in BD-associated uveitis, have been published. However, it was used with success in case series [37–39] and in a recent retrospective study. In this study, 10 out of 11 patients showed complete resolution of inflammation by 4 weeks [40]. Although more complete evidence is needed, particularly in the long-term efficacy and its use as a first-line therapy [41, 42], numerous publications suggest that infliximab represents an important therapeutic advancement in BD-associated uveitis. A therapeutic algorithm is proposed in figure 1.

Spondyloarthropathies and B27-Associated Uveitis

Uveitis is a well-known extra-rheumatologic manifestation of spondylarthropathies (including ankylosing spondylitis, AS, and psoriatic arthritis). A single

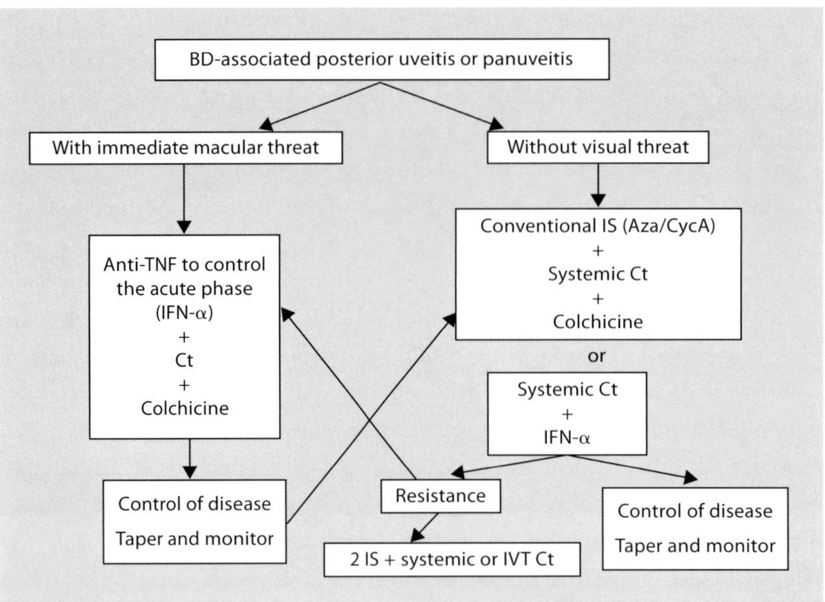

Fig. 1. Proposed algorithm for the treatment of BD-associated uveitis with posterior segment involvement. Ct = Corticosteroids; IS = immunosuppressive agents; Aza = azathioprine; CycA = cyclosporin A.

infusion of infliximab may be effective in treating an acute uveitis attack, but does not seem to affect disease recurrence [43]. In this indication, anti-TNF-α usefulness seems to be limited given that acute anterior uveitis generally responds to intensive corticosteroid therapy. A minority of cases could be managed with anti-TNF-α agents for chronic ocular complications which include posterior segment involvement or chronic disease refractory to conventional therapy [44]. The main interest of anti-TNF-α agents in this indication lies in preventing uveitis relapses. The effect of anti-TNF-α agents on anterior uveitis relapses in AS was analyzed in one large retrospective study [45] and in one meta-analysis of four clinical trials, three of which were placebo-controlled, randomized trials [21]. The retrospective study suggested that infliximab and adalimumab reduced the rate of uveitis, while the frequency of uveitis in patients with AS treated with etanercept remained unchanged [45]. In the meta-analysis, infliximab and etanercept therapies seem to reduce the incidence of uveitis even though infliximab appeared to be more effective than etanercept. However, the differences between infliximab and etanercept did not reach statistical significance ($p = 0.08$). Adalimumab was evaluated in a prospective open-label study showing its efficacy to prevent uveitis relapses in AS [46]. Hence, the use of an anti-TNF-α antibody should be considered first rather than using a soluble TNF receptor, in spondyloarthritis patients with a history of uveitis.

Juvenile Idiopathic Arthritis

Juvenile idiopathic arthritis (JIA) is a disease of unknown etiology that begins before the age of 16 years and persists for at least 6 weeks. JIA is a clinically heterogeneous group of diseases. The classification scheme developed by the International League of Associations of Rheumatologists in 2001 differentiates seven subtypes of JIA [47]. The risk of uveitis is highest in oligoarticular onset and extended oligoarticular forms [48]. The medical treatment of uveitis is challenging. Systemic corticosteroid therapy is often required, and immunomodulatory therapy is often needed in order to preserve visual acuity and to prevent significant morbidity of chronic steroid administration. Anti-TNF-α agents have been used with positive results. Although one previous study reported that etanercept had some efficacy in the treatment of chronic uveitis in children, subsequent studies failed to demonstrate a benefit [49]. A randomized placebo-controlled study of etanercept in patients with uveitis found no evidence of efficacy [16]. Furthermore, data from the German etanercept registry [50] showed insufficient control of uveitis by etanercept, whereas arthritis was well controlled. Multiple studies describe the efficacy of infliximab and adalimumab in JIA-associated uveitis [19, 51–54]. Recently, a prospective comparative study between infliximab and adalimumab in 33 children with refractory chronic uveitis (22 children with JIA) has been published. This study, without randomization, suggests that adalimumab is as efficacious as infliximab in a short-term period (31 of 33 children achieved complete remission), but maintains in remission for a longer period and with a higher rate. At 40 months, 9 (60%) of 15 children receiving adalimumab compared to 3 (18.8%) of 16 children receiving infliximab were still on remission ($p < 0.02$) [25]. This suggests the potential superiority of adalimumab in JIA-associated uveitis as previously hypothesized [55]. As in HLA-B27-associated uveitis, the use of infliximab and adalimumab should be considered first rather than using etanercept, in JIA patients with a history of uveitis.

Sarcoidosis

The first study mentioning successful anti-TNF-α use in steroid-resistant sarcoidosis was published in 2001 [56]. However, a placebo-controlled randomized study conducted to evaluate the safety and effectiveness of infliximab in subjects with chronic pulmonary sarcoidosis has not produced the expected results [57, 58]. Another randomized placebo-controlled study suggests that infliximab may be beneficial in the treatment of extrapulmonary sarcoidosis in patients already receiving corticosteroids, but authors found no improvement in patients with ocular disease who received infliximab [59]. Nevertheless, infliximab appears to be effective in ocular sarcoidosis, although data are limited to a case series [59] and to cases reports [25, 60, 61]. However, it is quite necessary to take into account the fact that sarcoidosis is underdiagnosed and a number of presumed, probable or possible sarcoid uveitis are labeled 'idiopathic' and may respond to anti-TNF-α [23]. Etanercept did not appear effective [17]. Adalimumab was successfully used recently in patients with uveitis and papillitis [62].

Uveitis Associated with Other Conditions

Few isolated cases of refractory Vogt-Koyanagi-Harada disease treated with infliximab were published with encouraging results [63–65]. Furthermore, infliximab was also used in pediatric forms [66] and adalimumab was used in a refractory case [67]. Successful use of infliximab in sympathetic ophthalmia has been reported in a few case reports [68–70]. Variable results induced by infliximab have been observed in birdshot chorioretinopathy [60, 61, 65, 71], in multifocal choroiditis [60, 72], and in idiopathic retinal vasculitis, aneurysm, and neuroretinitis syndrome [73]. Infliximab was used in a patient with refractory serpiginous choroiditis with a good clinical outcome. However, this patient died of disseminated tuberculosis (TB) after treatment [74]. Infliximab was also beneficial in patients with idiopathic refractory uveitis [51, 60, 75, 76] and diffuse subretinal fibrosis syndrome [77]. Etanercept has no significant efficacy over placebo in preventing relapses of idiopathic uveitis [15]. Adalimumab was able to control ocular inflammation in idiopathic refractory uveitis [25, 37].

Adverse Events

Anti-TNF-α agents in patients with uveitis seem well tolerated except for one study [60], but long-term studies on safety in uveitis are still missing. Safety profile of anti-TNF-α agents in rheumatoid arthritis is well known, and data could be extrapolated by taking into account the fact that differences between safety profiles according to different diseases were noted.

Infections

Anti-TNF-α agents carry a specifically increased risk of TB, usually reactivations of latent disease [78] but also primary infection. Important differences in the risk of latent TB reactivation exist, with the risk being higher with infliximab and adalimumab than with etanercept [79, 80]. Screening for latent TB and prophylactic anti-TB for all those found positive is recommended for all patients planning to initiate therapy with anti-TNF-α agents. The role of new screening tests for TB (Quantiferon and T-spot) has not been fully validated in this indication even though they can improve sensitivity in the immunosuppressed host and specificity in patients who have received Bacille Calmette-Guérin immunization. Finally, clinical similarities between ocular TB and other uveitis entities, such as choroidal TB and serpiginous choroidopathy [74], highlight the importance of ruling out TB in all refractory uveitis before initiating an anti-TNF-α therapy. Various and severe non-TB opportunistic infections, especially those with intracellular micro-organisms, may develop in patients receiving anti-TNF-α treatment. Furthermore, infliximab and adalimumab rather than soluble TNF receptor therapy and steroid use >10 mg/day were reported to be independently associated with opportunistic infections [81]. The safety profile of anti-TNF-α agents in the setting of hepatitis C infection seems to be acceptable, even though close monitoring of serum amino-transaminases should be performed during treatment. However, for patients with hepatitis B, concomitant anti-viral treatment would be recommended [82].

Demyelination

Several demyelinating and neurologic events, including exacerbations of pre-existing multiple sclerosis and optic neuritis, were reported implicating infliximab, adalimumab and etanercept [83–87]. Hence, anti-TNF-α therapy should not be given when there is a clear history of multiple sclerosis; it should be used with caution for other demyelinating diseases, and withdrawn if demyelination occurs [82]. Furthermore, it seems appropriate to recommend brain MR imaging to exclude multiple sclerosis in patients with intermediate uveitis and retinal vasculitis before receiving anti-TNF-α therapy.

Others

There is no conclusive evidence for an increase in risk of solid tumors or lymphoproliferative diseases with anti-TNF-α agents, although vigilance is required [82]. Development of antinuclear antibodies and autoantibodies against double-stranded DNA has previously been reported in response to etanercept, infliximab and adalimumab, but may be more common with infliximab. However, 'full-blown' anti-TNF-induced lupus or vasculitis is rare [88]. Injection site reactions occur with the use of etanercept, adalimumab, certolizumab pegol and golimumab. Infliximab can induce the formation of neutralizing antibodies, resulting in loss of efficacy and the appearance of infusion reactions [89]. Furthermore, antibodies have been also reported, to a lesser extent, against adalimumab, certolizumab pegol and golimumab. In most of cases, a conventional immunosuppressive agent such as methotrexate is associated with the treatment in order to prevent this complication. New onset and worsening of congestive heart failure have been reported, hence anti-TNF-α agents should not be initiated in patients with moderate and severe cardiac failure and should be used with caution in patients with mild cardiac failure [82]. Hematological complications associated with anti-TNF-α therapy are rare.

Paradoxical Adverse Events

A rare and paradoxical adverse event is the development of sarcoidosis during treatment with infliximab, adalimumab and etanercept [90–93]. Paradoxical occurrence of psoriasis has also been reported [94]. The issue of whether anti-TNF agents cause ocular inflammation remains a matter of debate [95]. There are several case reports of uveitis developing in patients treated with anti-TNF-α therapy. Most cases have been reported with etanercept [96–102]. However, as etanercept was shown to be less effective than anti-TNF-α antibodies to prevent and to control uveitis, does it induce uveitis or does it only fail to prevent their occurrence? Nonetheless, Lim et al. [95] reported 26 cases of uveitis presumably associated with anti-TNF-α in which no known condition predisposing to uveitis was identified. However, authors conceded that there was limited information available on the clinical diagnosis. Especially in the case of granulomatous uveitis, occurrence might be due to a potential sarcoidosis associated with anti-TNF-α [90]. Therefore, even though more data are required, switch for infliximab and adalimumab may be warranted when a patient develops uveitis during etanercept therapy.

Ocular Surgery

The French Rheumatology Society recommends interrupting TNF-α therapy for two half-lives before surgery in a sterile setting such as cataract surgery. However, very few data concerning cataract surgery in uveitis patients under anti-TNF-α are available, and the potential benefit of preventing postoperative infections by stopping treatment should be balanced against the risk of a perioperative intraocular inflammation recurrence. Up to now, few patients receiving infliximab for BD-associated uveitis were reported. Cataract surgery was performed without any complications 1 and 4 weeks after anti-TNF-α agents [103–105].

'Switching' Anti-TNF-α Agents

Switching between anti-TNF-α agents may be necessary. Efficacy and safety of switching between anti-TNF-α therapies have been well studied in other diseases. There is little evidence that 'switching' helps to gain or maintain uveitis remission. Nonetheless, case reports and a case series concerning BD and JIA-associated uveitis suggest that switching infliximab to adalimumab was successful to control uveitis in case of inefficacy [52, 106, 107], in case of intolerance or to avoid repeated injections [34, 108].

Future Directions

A topically applied TNF-α inhibitor single-chain antibody named ESBA105 is under development for patients suffering from acute anterior uveitis. In a prospective series of 5 patients with refractory uveitic macular edema, intravitreal adalimumab was not successful in reducing central retinal thickness and improving visual acuity [109]. In this study, no ocular or systemic adverse events were observed. Nevertheless, contradictory results about safety of intravitreal adalimumab injections have been published [109–112]. Intravitreal infliximab injections were not tested up to now in uveitis treatment. However, contradictory results concerning its safety have been published [113–115]. Further studies focusing on the concentration and toxic effects of intravitreal injections of anti-TNF-α agents are necessary, although their efficacy remains uncertain.

Conclusions

Anti-TNF-α agents are widely used for the treatment of noninfectious uveitis even though it remains mostly an off-label use. The lack of evidence from randomized controlled studies in the uveitis area limits a rationale choice and initiation time of anti-TNF-α therapy, the molecule type and duration of treatment. Furthermore, this is a rapidly changing field with new data emerging regularly. Nevertheless, to the best of our knowledge, a few issues may be addressed.

Which one? There are no head-to-head randomized comparative studies comparing efficacy of anti-TNF-α agents in uveitis area. Nevertheless, etanercept should not be used in case of uveitis. Adalimumab might appear as the most favorable anti-TNF-α agents because of its facility of administration, its low rate of neutralizing antibodies induction and its possible superior efficacy to maintain in remission chronic refractory uveitis in children. One limitation with adalimumab may be its lower efficacy on different rheumatic conditions, compared with infliximab. As golimumab requires less frequent injections, it might have potential application in uveitis area if its efficacy and its side effect profile do not differ from the first-generation agents.

When? After ruling out ocular TB and latent TB, anti-TNF-α agents could be used as a third-line treatment in chronic refractory uveitis as maintenance therapy. However, in rescue therapy, infliximab infusion may be considered particularly in BD-associated uveitis, and anti-TNF-α maintenance therapy might be considered earlier to avoid drug-induced side effects particularly in children.

How Long? Currently, no response is available. However, anti-TNF-α therapy seems to be well tolerated with a relatively few side effects. Given collective clinical experience in uveitis and other conditions, switching between anti-TNF-α therapies appears to be efficacious and safe in cases of primary or secondary failure permitting to prolong their use. Compared with other biologic agents such as IFN-α, treatment with anti-TNF-α induces remission, but relapses occur very frequently after discontinuation.

References

1 Beutler B, Greenwald D, Hulmes JD, Chang M, Pan YC, Mathison J, Ulevitch R, Cerami A: Identity of tumour necrosis factor and the macrophage-secreted factor cachectin. Nature 1985;316:552–554.

2 Heiligenhaus A, Thurau S, Hennig M, Grajewski RS, Wildner G: Anti-inflammatory treatment of uveitis with biologicals: new treatment options that reflect pathogenetic knowledge of the disease. Graefes Arch Clin Exp Ophthalmol 2010;248:1531–1551.

3 Roach DR, Bean AG, Demangel C, France MP, Briscoe H, Britton WJ: TNF regulates chemokine induction essential for cell recruitment, granuloma formation, and clearance of mycobacterial infection. J Immunol 2002;168:4620–4627.

4 de Vos AF, Klaren VN, Kijlstra A: Expression of multiple cytokines and IL-1RA in the uvea and retina during endotoxin-induced uveitis in the rat. Invest Ophthalmol Vis Sci 1994;35:3873–3883.

5 de Vos AF, van Haren MA, Verhagen C, Hoekzema R, Kijlstra A: Kinetics of intraocular tumor necrosis factor and interleukin-6 in endotoxin-induced uveitis in the rat. Invest Ophthalmol Vis Sci 1994;35:1100–1106.

6 Woon MD, Kaplan HJ, Bora NS: Kinetics of cytokine production in experimental autoimmune anterior uveitis (EAAU). Curr Eye Res 1998;17:955–961.

7 Okada AA, Sakai J, Usui M, Mizuguchi J: Intraocular cytokine quantification of experimental autoimmune uveoretinitis in rats. Ocul Immunol Inflamm 1998;6:111–120.

8 Rosenbaum JT, Howes Jr EL, Rubin RM, Samples JR: Ocular inflammatory effects of intravitreally-injected tumor necrosis factor. Am J Pathol 1988;133:47–53.

9 De Vos AF, Van Haren MA, Verhagen C, Hoekzema R, Kijlstra A: Tumour necrosis factor-induced uveitis in the Lewis rat is associated with intraocular interleukin 6 production. Exp Eye Res 1995;60:199–207.

10 Perez-Guijo V, Santos-Lacomba M, Sanchez-Hernandez M, Castro-Villegas Mdel C, Gallardo-Galera JM, Collantes-Estevez E: Tumour necrosis factor-alpha levels in aqueous humour and serum from patients with uveitis: the involvement of HLA-B27. Curr Med Res Opin 2004;20:155–157.

11 Sakaguchi M, Sugita S, Sagawa K, Itoh K, Mochizuki M: Cytokine production by T cells infiltrating in the eye of uveitis patients. Jpn J Ophthalmol 1998;42:262–268.

12 Kasner L, Chan CC, Whitcup SM, Gery I: The paradoxical effect of tumor necrosis factor alpha (TNF-alpha) in endotoxin-induced uveitis. Invest Ophthalmol Vis Sci 1993;34:2911–2917.

13 Rosenbaum JT, Boney RS: Failure to inhibit endotoxin-induced uveitis with antibodies that neutralize tumor necrosis factor. Reg Immunol 1993;5:299–303.

14 Scallon B, Cai A, Solowski N, Rosenberg A, Song XY, Shealy D, Wagner C: Binding and functional comparisons of two types of tumor necrosis factor antagonists. J Pharmacol Exp Ther 2002;301:418–426.

15 Foster CS, Tufail F, Waheed NK, Chu D, Miserocchi E, Baltatzis S, Vredeveld CM: Efficacy of etanercept in preventing relapse of uveitis controlled by methotrexate. Arch Ophthalmol 2003;121:437–440.

16 Smith JA, Thompson DJ, Whitcup SM, Suhler E, Clarke G, Smith S, Robinson M, Kim J, Barron KS: A randomized, placebo-controlled, double-masked clinical trial of etanercept for the treatment of uveitis associated with juvenile idiopathic arthritis. Arthritis Rheum 2005;53:18–23.

17 Baughman RP, Lower EE, Bradley DA, Raymond LA, Kaufman A: Etanercept for refractory ocular sarcoidosis: results of a double-blind randomized trial. Chest 2005;128:1062–1047.

18 Galor A, Perez VL, Hammel JP, Lowder CY: Differential effectiveness of etanercept and infliximab in the treatment of ocular inflammation. Ophthalmology 2006;113:2317–2323.

19 Foeldvari I, Nielsen S, Kummerle-Deschner J, Espada G, Horneff G, Bica B, Olivieri AN, Wierk A, Saurenmann RK: Tumor necrosis factor-alpha blocker in treatment of juvenile idiopathic arthritis-associated uveitis refractory to second-line agents: results of a multinational survey. J Rheumatol 2007;34:1146–1150.

20 Tynjala P, Lindahl P, Honkanen V, Lahdenne P, Kotaniemi K: Infliximab and etanercept in the treatment of chronic uveitis associated with refractory juvenile idiopathic arthritis. Ann Rheum Dis 2007;66:548–550.

21 Braun J, Baraliakos X, Listing J, Sieper J: Decreased incidence of anterior uveitis in patients with ankylosing spondylitis treated with the anti-tumor necrosis factor agents infliximab and etanercept. Arthritis Rheum 2005;52:2447–2451.

22 Imrie FR, Dick AD: Biologics in the treatment of uveitis. Curr Opin Ophthalmol 2007;18:481–486.

23 Sharma SM, Nestel AR, Lee RW, Dick AD: Clinical review: anti-TNFalpha therapies in uveitis: perspective on 5 years of clinical experience. Ocul Immunol Inflamm 2009;17:403–414.

24 Neri P, Zucchi M, Allegri P, Lettieri M, Mariotti C, Giovannini A: Adalimumab (Humira): a promising monoclonal anti-tumor necrosis factor alpha in ophthalmology. Int Ophthalmol 2011;31:165–173.

25 Simonini G, Taddio A, Cattalini M, Caputo R, De Libero C, Naviglio S, Bresci C, Lorusso M, Lepore L, Cimaz R: Prevention of flare recurrences in childhood-refractory chronic uveitis: an open-label comparative study of adalimumab versus infliximab. Arthritis Care Res (Hoboken) 2011;63:612–618.

26 Cordero-Coma M, Salom D, Diaz-Llopis M, Lopez-Prats MJ, Calleja S: Golimumab for uveitis. Ophthalmology 2011;118:1892, e1893–e1894.

27 Sfikakis PP, Markomichelakis N, Alpsoy E, Assaad-Khalil S, Bodaghi B, Gul A, Ohno S, Pipitone N, Schirmer M, Stanford M, Wechsler B, Zouboulis C, Kaklamanis P, Yazici H: Anti-TNF therapy in the management of Behcet's disease–review and basis for recommendations. Rheumatology (Oxford) 2007;46: 736–741.

28 Melikoglu M, Fresko I, Mat C, Ozyazgan Y, Gogus F, Yurdakul S, Hamuryudan V, Yazici H: Short-term trial of etanercept in Behcet's disease: a double blind, placebo controlled study. J Rheumatol 2005;32: 98–105.

29 Sfikakis PP, Theodossiadis PG, Katsiari CG, Kaklamanis P, Markomichelakis NN: Effect of infliximab on sight-threatening panuveitis in Behcet's disease. Lancet 2001;358:295–296.

30 Arida A, Fragiadaki K, Giavri E, Sfikakis PP: Anti-TNF agents for Behcet's Disease: analysis of published data on 369 patients. Semin Arthritis Rheum 2011;41:61–70.

31 Hatemi G, Silman A, Bang D, Bodaghi B, Chamberlain AM, Gul A, Houman MH, Kotter I, Olivieri I, Salvarani C, Sfikakis PP, Siva A, Stanford MR, Stubiger N, Yurdakul S, Yazici H: EULAR recommendations for the management of Behcet disease. Ann Rheum Dis 2008;67:1656–1662.

32 Hatemi G, Silman A, Bang D, Bodaghi B, Chamberlain AM, Gul A, Houman MH, Kotter I, Olivieri I, Salvarani C, Sfikakis PP, Siva A, Stanford MR, Stubiger N, Yurdakul S, Yazici H: Management of Behcet disease: a systematic literature review for the European League Against Rheumatism evidence-based recommendations for the management of Behcet disease. Ann Rheum Dis 2009;68:1528–1534.

33 Gueudry J, Wechsler B, Terrada C, Gendron G, Cassoux N, Fardeau C, Lehoang P, Piette JC, Bodaghi B: Long-term efficacy and safety of low-dose interferon alpha2a therapy in severe uveitis associated with Behcet disease. Am J Ophthalmol 2008;146:837–844, e831.

34 Mushtaq B, Saeed T, Situnayake RD, Murray PI: Adalimumab for sight-threatening uveitis in Behcet's disease. Eye (Lond) 2007;21:824–825.

35 Ohno S, Nakamura S, Hori S, Shimakawa M, Kawashima H, Mochizuki M, Sugita S, Ueno S, Yoshizaki K, Inaba G: Efficacy, safety, and pharmacokinetics of multiple administration of infliximab in Behcet's disease with refractory uveoretinitis. J Rheumatol 2004;31:1362–1368.

36 Markomichelakis N, Delicha E, Masselos S, Fragiadaki K, Kaklamanis P, Sfikakis PP: A single infliximab infusion vs corticosteroids for acute panuveitis attacks in Behcet's disease: a comparative 4-week study. Rheumatology (Oxford) 2011;50:593–597.

37 Diaz-Llopis M, Garcia-Delpech S, Salom D, Udaondo P, Hernandez-Garfella M, Bosch-Morell F, Quijada A, Romero FJ: Adalimumab therapy for refractory uveitis: a pilot study. J Ocul Pharmacol Ther 2008;24:351–361.

38 Callejas-Rubio JL, Sanchez-Cano D, Serrano JL, Ortego-Centeno N: Adalimumab therapy for refractory uveitis: a pilot study. J Ocul Pharmacol Ther 2008;24:613–614, author reply 614.

39 van Laar JA, Missotten T, van Daele PL, Jamnitski A, Baarsma GS, van Hagen PM: Adalimumab: a new modality for Behcet's disease? Ann Rheum Dis 2007;66:565–566.

40 Bawazeer A, Raffa LH, Nizamuddin SH: Clinical experience with adalimumab in the treatment of ocular Behcet disease. Ocul Immunol Inflamm 2010;18:226–232.

41 Yamada Y, Sugita S, Tanaka H, Kamoi K, Kawaguchi T, Mochizuki M: Comparison of infliximab versus ciclosporin during the initial 6-month treatment period in Behcet disease. Br J Ophthalmol 2010;94: 284–288.

42 Lee RW, Dick AD: Treat early and embrace the evidence in favour of anti-TNF-alpha therapy for Behcet's uveitis. Br J Ophthalmol 2010;94:269–270.

43 El-Shabrawi Y, Hermann J: Anti-tumor necrosis factor-alpha therapy with infliximab as an alternative to corticosteroids in the treatment of human leukocyte antigen B27-associated acute anterior uveitis. Ophthalmology 2002;109:2342–2346.

44 El-Shabrawi Y, Hermann J: Case series of selective anti-tumor necrosis factor alpha therapy using infliximab in patients with nonresponsive chronic HLA-B27-associated anterior uveitis: comment on the articles by Brandt et al. Arthritis Rheum 2002;46:2821–2822, author reply 2822–2824.

45 Guignard S, Gossec L, Salliot C, Ruyssen-Witrand A, Luc M, Duclos M, Dougados M: Efficacy of tumour necrosis factor blockers in reducing uveitis flares in patients with spondylarthropathy: a retrospective study. Ann Rheum Dis 2006;65:1631–1634.

46 Rudwaleit M, Rodevand E, Holck P, Vanhoof J, Kron M, Kary S, Kupper H: Adalimumab effectively reduces the rate of anterior uveitis flares in patients with active ankylosing spondylitis: results of a prospective open-label study. Ann Rheum Dis 2009;68: 696–701.

47 Petty RE, Southwood TR, Manners P, Baum J, Glass DN, Goldenberg J, He X, Maldonado-Cocco J, Orozco-Alcala J, Prieur AM, Suarez-Almazor ME, Woo P: International League of Associations for Rheumatology classification of juvenile idiopathic arthritis: second revision, Edmonton, 2001. J Rheumatol 2004;31:390–392.

48 Marvillet I, Terrada C, Quartier P, Quoc EB, Bodaghi B, Prieur AM: Ocular threat in juvenile idiopathic arthritis. Joint Bone Spine 2009;76:383–388.

49 Reiff A, Takei S, Sadeghi S, Stout A, Shaham B, Bernstein B, Gallagher K, Stout T: Etanercept therapy in children with treatment-resistant uveitis. Arthritis Rheum 2001;44:1411–1415.

50 Schmeling H, Horneff G: Etanercept and uveitis in patients with juvenile idiopathic arthritis. Rheumatology (Oxford) 2005;44:1008–1011.

51 Saurenmann RK, Levin AV, Rose JB, Parker S, Rabinovitch T, Tyrrell PN, Feldman BM, Laxer RM, Schneider R, Silverman ED: Tumour necrosis factor alpha inhibitors in the treatment of childhood uveitis. Rheumatology (Oxford) 2006;45:982–989.

52 Biester S, Deuter C, Michels H, Haefner R, Kuemmerle-Deschner J, Doycheva D, Zierhut M: Adalimumab in the therapy of uveitis in childhood. Br J Ophthalmol 2007;91:319–324.

53 Vazquez-Cobian LB, Flynn T, Lehman TJ: Adalimumab therapy for childhood uveitis. J Pediatr 2006;149:572–575.

54 Gallagher M, Quinones K, Cervantes-Castaneda RA, Yilmaz T, Foster CS: Biological response modifier therapy for refractory childhood uveitis. Br J Ophthalmol 2007;91:1341–1344.

55 Mansour AM: Adalimumab in the therapy of uveitis in childhood. Br J Ophthalmol 2007;91:274–276.

56 Baughman RP, Lower EE: Infliximab for refractory sarcoidosis. Sarcoidosis Vasc Diffuse Lung Dis 2001;18:70–74.

57 Bargagli E, Olivieri C, Rottoli P: Cytokine modulators in the treatment of sarcoidosis. Rheumatol Int 2011;31:1539–1544.

58 Rossman MD, Newman LS, Baughman RP, Teirstein A, Weinberger SE, Miller Jr W, Sands BE: A double-blinded, randomized, placebo-controlled trial of infliximab in subjects with active pulmonary sarcoidosis. Sarcoidosis Vasc Diffuse Lung Dis 2006;23: 201–208.

59 Judson MA, Baughman RP, Costabel U, Flavin S, Lo KH, Kavuru MS, Drent M: Efficacy of infliximab in extrapulmonary sarcoidosis: results from a randomised trial. Eur Respir J 2008;31:1189–1196.

60 Suhler EB, Smith JR, Wertheim MS, Lauer AK, Kurz DE, Pickard TD, Rosenbaum JT: A prospective trial of infliximab therapy for refractory uveitis: preliminary safety and efficacy outcomes. Arch Ophthalmol 2005;123:903–912.

61 Lindstedt EW, Baarsma GS, Kuijpers RW, van Hagen PM: Anti-TNF-alpha therapy for sight threatening uveitis. Br J Ophthalmol 2005;89:533–536.

62 Lahmer T, Knopf A, Lanzl I, Heemann U, Thuermel K: Using TNF-alpha antagonist adalimumab for treatment for multisystem sarcoidosis: a case study. Rheumatol Int 2011, Epub ahead of print.

63 Niccoli L, Nannini C, Cassara E, Gini G, Lenzetti I, Cantini F: Efficacy of infliximab therapy in two patients with refractory Vogt-Koyanagi-Harada disease. Br J Ophthalmol 2009;93:1553–1554.

64 Wang Y, Gaudio PA: Infliximab therapy for 2 patients with Vogt-Koyanagi-Harada syndrome. Ocul Immunol Inflamm 2008;16:167–171.

65 Baughman RP, Bradley DA, Lower EE: Infliximab in chronic ocular inflammation. Int J Clin Pharmacol Ther 2005;43:7–11.

66 Khalifa YM, Bailony MR, Acharya NR: Treatment of pediatric Vogt-Koyanagi-Harada syndrome with infliximab. Ocul Immunol Inflamm 2010;18:218–222.

67 Diaz Llopis M, Amselem L, Romero FJ, Garcia-Delpech S, Hernandez ML: Adalimumab therapy for Vogt-Koyanagi-Harada syndrome (in Spanish). Arch Soc Esp Oftalmol 2007;82:131–132.

68 Ziahosseini K, Newman WD: Challenges of managing sympathetic ophthalmia in a young child and the role of infliximab. J Pediatr Ophthalmol Strabismus 2011;48:e34–e36.

69 Menghini M, Frimmel SA, Windisch R, Meier FM: Efficacy of infliximab therapy in two patients with sympathetic ophthalmia. Klin Monbl Augenheilkd 2011;228:362–363.

70 Gupta SR, Phan IT, Suhler EB: Successful treatment of refractory sympathetic ophthalmia in a child with infliximab. Arch Ophthalmol 2011;129:250–252.

71 Petropoulos IK, Vaudaux JD, Guex-Crosier Y: Anti-TNF-alpha therapy in patients with chronic non-infectious uveitis: the experience of Jules Gonin Eye Hospital. Klin Monbl Augenheilkd 2008;225:457–461.

72 Benitez-del-Castillo JM, Martinez-de-la-Casa JM, Pato-Cour E, Mendez-Fernandez R, Lopez-Abad C, Matilla M, Garcia-Sanchez J: Long-term treatment of refractory posterior uveitis with anti-TNFalpha (infliximab). Eye (Lond) 2005;19:841–845.

73 Cheema RA, Al-Askar E, Cheema HR: Infliximab therapy for idiopathic retinal vasculitis, aneurysm, and neuroretinitis syndrome. J Ocul Pharmacol Ther 2011;27:407–410.

74 Cordero-Coma M, Benito MF, Hernandez AM, Antolin SC, Ruiz JM: Serpiginous choroiditis. Ophthalmology 2008;115:1633, e1631–e1632.

75 Murphy CC, Greiner K, Plskova J, Duncan L, Frost A, Isaacs JD, Rebello P, Waldmann H, Hale G, Forrester JV, Dick AD: Neutralizing tumor necrosis factor activity leads to remission in patients with refractory noninfectious posterior uveitis. Arch Ophthalmol 2004;122:845–851.

76 Bodaghi B, Bui Quoc E, Wechsler B, Tran TH, Cassoux N, Le Thi Huong D, Chosidow O, Herson S, Piette JC, LeHoang P: Therapeutic use of infliximab in sight threatening uveitis: retrospective analysis of efficacy, safety, and limiting factors. Ann Rheum Dis 2005;64:962–964.

77 Adan A, Sanmarti R, Bures A, Casaroli-Marano RP: Successful treatment with infliximab in a patient with diffuse subretinal fibrosis syndrome. Am J Ophthalmol 2007;143:533–534.

78 Keane J, Gershon S, Wise RP, Mirabile-Levens E, Kasznica J, Schwieterman WD, Siegel JN, Braun MM: Tuberculosis associated with infliximab, a tumor necrosis factor alpha-neutralizing agent. N Engl J Med 2001;345:1098–1104.

79 Dixon WG, Hyrich KL, Watson KD, Lunt M, Galloway J, Ustianowski A, Symmons DP: Drug-specific risk of tuberculosis in patients with rheumatoid arthritis treated with anti-TNF therapy: results from the British Society for Rheumatology Biologics Register (BSRBR). Ann Rheum Dis 2009;69:522–528.

80 Tubach F, Salmon D, Ravaud P, Allanore Y, Goupille P, Breban M, Pallot-Prades B, Pouplin S, Sacchi A, Chichemanian RM, Bretagne S, Emilie D, Lemann M, Lortholary O, Mariette X: Risk of tuberculosis is higher with anti-tumor necrosis factor monoclonal antibody therapy than with soluble tumor necrosis factor receptor therapy: the three-year prospective French Research Axed on Tolerance of Biotherapies registry. Arthritis Rheum 2009;60:1884–1894.

81 Salmon-Ceron D, Tubach F, Lortholary O, Chosidow O, Bretagne S, Nicolas N, Cuillerier E, Fautrel B, Michelet C, Morel J, Puechal X, Wendling D, Lemann M, Ravaud P, Mariette X: Drug-specific risk of non-tuberculosis opportunistic infections in patients receiving anti-TNF therapy reported to the 3-year prospective French RATIO registry. Ann Rheum Dis 2011;70:616–623.

82 Ding T, Ledingham J, Luqmani R, Westlake S, Hyrich K, Lunt M, Kiely P, Bukhari M, Abernethy R, Bosworth A, Ostor A, Gadsby K, McKenna F, Finney D, Dixey J, Deighton C: BSR and BHPR rheumatoid arthritis guidelines on safety of anti-TNF therapies. Rheumatology (Oxford) 2010;49:2217–2219.

83 Simsek I, Erdem H, Pay S, Sobaci G, Dinc A: Optic neuritis occurring with anti-tumour necrosis factor alpha therapy. Ann Rheum Dis 2007;66:1255–1258.

84 Cunningham ET, Zierhut M: TNF inhibitors for uveitis: balancing efficacy and safety. Ocul Immunol Inflamm 2010;18:421–423.

85 Stubgen JP: Tumor necrosis factor-alpha antagonists and neuropathy. Muscle Nerve 2008;37:281–292.

86 Solomon AJ, Spain RI, Kruer MC, Bourdette D: Inflammatory neurological disease in patients treated with tumor necrosis factor alpha inhibitors. Mult Scler 2011;17:1472–1487.

87 Bensouda-Grimaldi L, Mulleman D, Valat JP, Autret-Leca E: Adalimumab-associated multiple sclerosis. J Rheumatol 2007;34:239–240, discussion 240.

88 Williams EL, Gadola S, Edwards CJ: Anti-TNF-induced lupus. Rheumatology (Oxford) 2009;48:716–720.

89 Pascual-Salcedo D, Plasencia C, Ramiro S, Nuno L, Bonilla G, Nagore D, Ruiz Del Agua A, Martinez A, Aarden L, Martin-Mola E, Balsa A: Influence of immunogenicity on the efficacy of long-term treatment with infliximab in rheumatoid arthritis. Rheumatology (Oxford) 2011;50:1445–1452.

90 Hashkes PJ, Shajrawi I: Sarcoid-related uveitis occurring during etanercept therapy. Clin Exp Rheumatol 2003;21:645–646.

91 Sturfelt G, Christensson B, Bynke G, Saxne T: Neurosarcoidosis in a patient with rheumatoid arthritis during treatment with infliximab. J Rheumatol 2007;34:2313–2314.

92 Daien CI, Monnier A, Claudepierre P, Constantin A, Eschard JP, Houvenagel E, Samimi M, Pavy S, Pertuiset E, Toussirot E, Combe B, Morel J: Sarcoid-like granulomatosis in patients treated with tumor necrosis factor blockers: 10 cases. Rheumatology (Oxford) 2009;48:883–886.

93 Louie GH, Chitkara P, Ward MM: Relapse of sarcoidosis upon treatment with etanercept. Ann Rheum Dis 2008;67:896–898.

94 Ko JM, Gottlieb AB, Kerbleski JF: Induction and exacerbation of psoriasis with TNF-blockade therapy: a review and analysis of 127 cases. J Dermatolog Treat 2009;20:100–108.

95 Lim LL, Fraunfelder FW, Rosenbaum JT: Do tumor necrosis factor inhibitors cause uveitis? A registry-based study. Arthritis Rheum 2007;56:3248–3252.

96 Cobo-Ibanez T, del Carmen Ordonez M, Munoz-Fernandez S, Madero-Prado R, Martin-Mola E: Do TNF-blockers reduce or induce uveitis? Rheumatology (Oxford) 2008;47:731–732.

97 Scrivo R, Spadaro A, Spinelli FR, Valesini G: Uveitis following the use of tumor necrosis factor alpha inhibitors: comment on the article by Lim et al. Arthritis Rheum 2008;58:1555–1556, author reply 1556–1557.

98 Kakkassery V, Mergler S, Pleyer U: Anti-TNF-alpha treatment: a possible promoter in endogenous uveitis? Observational report on six patients: occurrence of uveitis following etanercept treatment. Curr Eye Res 2010;35:751–756.

99 Reddy AR, Backhouse OC: Does etanercept induce uveitis? Br J Ophthalmol 2003;87:925.

100 Taban M, Dupps WJ, Mandell B, Perez VL: Etanercept (enbrel)-associated inflammatory eye disease: case report and review of the literature. Ocul Immunol Inflamm 2006;14:145–150.

101 Tiliakos AN, Tiliakos NA: Ocular inflammatory disease in patients with RA taking etanercept: is discontinuation of etanercept necessary? J Rheumatol 2003;30:2727.

102 Kaipiainen-Seppanen O, Leino M: Recurrent uveitis in a patient with juvenile spondyloarthropathy associated with tumour necrosis factor alpha inhibitors. Ann Rheum Dis 2003;62:88–89.

103 Handa T, Tsunekawa H, Zako M: Cataract surgery in Behcet's disease patients one week after infliximab administration. Case Report Ophthalmol 2011;2:176–178.

104 Sakai T, Kanetaka A, Noro T, Tsuneoka H: Intraocular surgery in patients receiving infliximab therapy for Behcet disease. Jpn J Ophthalmol 2010; 54:360–361.

105 Noda E, Yamanishi S, Shiraishi A, Ohashi Y: Cataract surgery under infliximab therapy in a patient with Behcet's disease. J Ocul Pharmacol Ther 2009;25:467–470.

106 Leccese P, Latanza L, D'Angelo S, Padula A, Olivieri I: Efficacy of switching to adalimumab in a patient with refractory uveitis of Behcet's disease to infliximab. Clin Exp Rheumatol 2011;29(suppl 67):S93.

107 Dhingra N, Morgan J, Dick AD: Switching biologic agents for uveitis. Eye (Lond) 2009;23:1868–1870.

108 Takase K, Ohno S, Ideguchi H, Uchio E, Takeno M, Ishigatsubo Y: Successful switching to adalimumab in an infliximab-allergic patient with severe Behcet disease-related uveitis. Rheumatol Int 2011;31:243–245.

109 Androudi S, Tsironi E, Kalogeropoulos C, Theodoridou A, Brazitikos P: Intravitreal adalimumab for refractory uveitis-related macular edema. Ophthalmology 2010;117:1612–1616.

110 Manzano RP, Peyman GA, Carvounis PE, Damico FM, Aguiar RG, Ioshimoto GL, Ventura DF, Cursino ST, Takahashi W: Toxicity of high-dose intravitreal adalimumab (Humira) in the rabbit. J Ocul Pharmacol Ther 2011;27:327–331.

111 Manzano RP, Peyman GA, Carvounis PE, Kivilcim M, Khan P, Chevez-Barrios P, Takahashi W: Ocular toxicity of intravitreous adalimumab (Humira) in the rabbit. Graefes Arch Clin Exp Ophthalmol 2008;246:907–911.

112 Tsilimbaris M, Diakonis VF, Naoumidi I, Charisis S, Kritikos I, Chatzithanasis G, Papadaki T, Plainis S: Evaluation of potential retinal toxicity of adalimumab (Humira). Graefes Arch Clin Exp Ophthalmol 2009;247:1119–1125.

113 Giganti M, Beer PM, Lemanski N, Hartman C, Schartman J, Falk N: Adverse events after intravitreal infliximab (Remicade). Retina 2010;30:71–80.

114 Theodossiadis PG, Liarakos VS, Sfikakis PP, Charonis A, Agrogiannis G, Kavantzas N, Vergados IA: Intravitreal administration of the anti-TNF monoclonal antibody infliximab in the rabbit. Graefes Arch Clin Exp Ophthalmol 2009;247:273–281.

115 Theodossiadis PG, Liarakos VS, Sfikakis PP, Vergados IA, Theodossiadis GP: Intravitreal administration of the anti-tumor necrosis factor agent infliximab for neovascular age-related macular degeneration. Am J Ophthalmol 2009;147:825–830, e821.

Bahram Bodaghi
Department of Ophthalmology, University of Paris VI, Pitié-Salpêtrière Hospital
47 Boulevard de L'Hôpital
FR–75013 Paris (France)
Tel. +33 1 42 16 32 02, E-Mail bahram.bodaghi@psl.aphp.fr

Miserocchi E, Modorati G, Foster CS (eds): New Treatments in Noninfectious Uveitis.
Dev Ophthalmol. Basel, Karger, 2012, vol 51, pp 79–89

New Biologic Drugs: Anti-Interleukin Therapy

Christoph Tappeiner[a] · Burkhard Möller[b] · Maren Hennig[c] · Arnd Heiligenhaus[c]

Departments of [a]Ophthalmology and [b]Rheumatology, Allergology and Immunology, Inselspital, University of Bern, Bern, Switzerland; [c]Department of Ophthalmology, St. Franziskus Hospital, Münster, and University of Essen, Essen, Germany

Abstract

Interleukins (ILs) are cytokines which are defined by their capability to convey information between leukocytes, in this way directing proliferation, activation, and migration and also regulation of the cells. Data from anti-IL treatments in systemic autoimmune diseases have shown these drugs to be beneficial and to have a satisfactory safety profile and tolerance. Recent publications of small case series suggest that several anti-IL drugs have considerable efficacy in treating otherwise refractory uveitis. Anti-IL therapy, therefore, might constitute an option for the treatment of uveitis resistant to corticosteroids, classical immunosuppressives, or tumor necrosis factor-α inhibitors. However, due to high costs and possible long-term risks, anti-IL agents should currently be reserved to selected uveitis patients and be administered only under close interdisciplinary monitoring.

Introduction

Background Information: Interleukins and Uveitis

The role of different cytokines and inflammatory pathways in the cascade of intraocular inflammation (fig. 1) has been investigated in experimental animal models. Endotoxin-induced uveitis (EIU) in mice or rats resembles acute anterior uveitis in humans [1, 2]. In EIU, ocular or systemic injection of lipopolysaccharide induces a nonautoimmune anterior uveitis characterized by a nonspecific, innate immune response involving monocytes, macrophages, and neutrophils [1, 3, 4]. In addition to tumor necrosis factor (TNF)-α, the proinflammatory cytokines interleukin (IL)-1 and IL-6 play a major role in the pathogenesis of the ocular inflammation in EIU [5–7].

Experimental autoimmune uveoretinitis (EAU) simulates the pathogenesis of autoimmune posterior uveitis in humans [8]. The intraocular inflammation in EAU

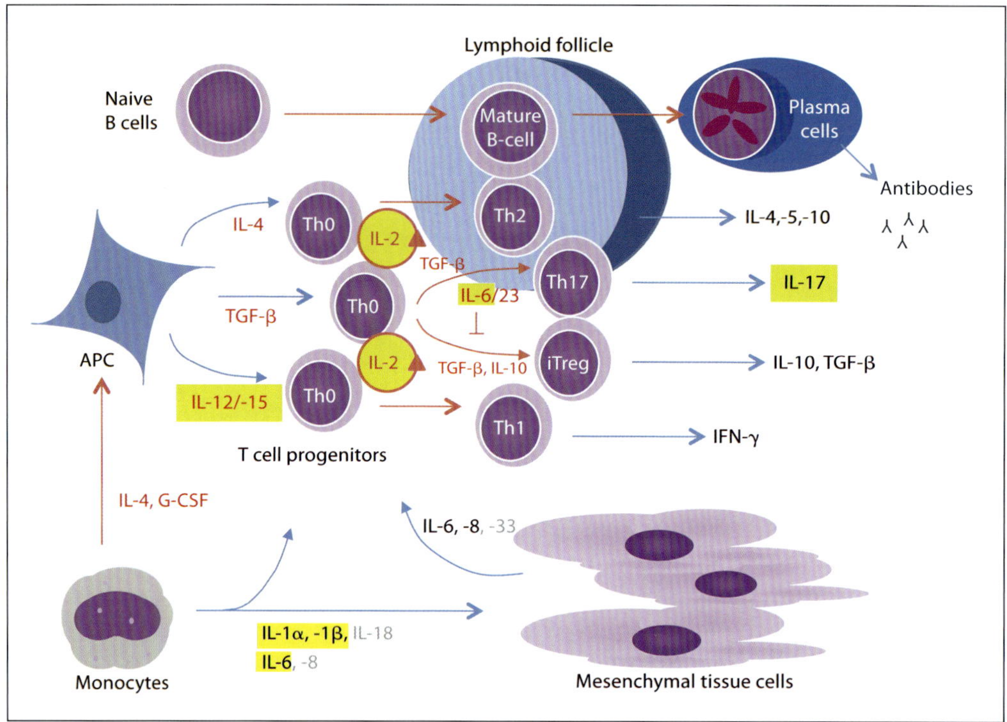

Fig. 1. Simplified scheme of the highly redundant IL system. The directly targeted ILs are highlighted with a yellow background. The adaptive immune system is represented by the antigen-presenting cells (APC) and its progenitors and by other mesenchymal tissue cells, such as endothelial cells and fibroblasts (bottom right). After maturation from monocytes (bottom left), dendritic cells constitute the main population of professional APC. Antigen presented by APC, costimulatory signaling, and ILs represent the signals important for T cell priming, and therefore, for directing and regulating adaptive immune processes in the secondary lymphoid organs, shown by the lymphoid follicle structure (top middle). This is also where Th2 cell-driven B cells develop from naïve to antibody-producing plasma cells. Regulatory T cells (Treg) are central in the inhibition of pathological immune processes. ILs required for the differentiation processes, for example of the Th cells, are shown in red, and the cell products are shown in black.

is mediated by antigen-specific CD4+ T cells, primarily of T helper (Th) cells type 1 and 17 (Th1, Th17) [9–12]. EAU can be induced in mice and rats by immunizing them with ocular antigens (e.g. S-antigen, interphotoreceptor-binding protein) or by adoptive transfer of uveitogenic T cells [13–17]. The inflammatory pathways of EAU are complex and have been reviewed in detail in previous publications [18–20]. After immunization, antigen-specific Th1 and Th17 cells are activated by antigen-presenting cells in the periphery, migrate to the ocular site, and overcome the local immune privilege. The expression of proinflammatory cytokines and chemokines by immune cells and resident cells attracts monocytes, macrophages, neutrophils, natural killer (NK) cells, natural killer T cells, and γδ-T cells and supports the development of a local nonspecific immune response, which results in tissue damage.

The uveitogenic effector responses involve different cytokine expression patterns (Th1: IL-1, IL-15, IL-2, IL-6, interferon (IFN)-γ, TNF-α; Th17: IL-17A, IL-17F, IL-21, IL-22, IL-6). Whereas IL-2 and IL-15 are important factors for the activation and survival of T cells and NK cells, IFN-γ and TNF-α represent important activators of cells of the innate immune system. IL-1 and IL-6 are essential for the induction of Th17 cells [21]. Ooi et al. [22] presented an overview of the levels of the various intraocular ILs that can be found in different forms of uveitis in humans, revealing elevated levels of IL-1β, IL-2, IL-6, IFN-γ and TNF-α, for example, in most cases of uveitis.

Although B cells and autoantibodies currently appear to play only a minor role in EAU induction, levels of Th2 cytokines (e.g. IL-4, IL-5, and IL-10), which are necessary for the activation, proliferation, and differentiation of B cells to antibody-producing plasma cells, are elevated [9, 23]. In juvenile idiopathic arthritis (JIA), the presence of anti-nuclear antibodies represents an important risk factor for the development of uveitis. However, the role of B cells in the pathogenesis of uveitis in humans is thus far not known.

What Is a Biologic Agent?

A biologic drug is defined as a protein produced by molecular recombinant DNA technology that is designed to have a therapeutic effect based on current understanding of the disease pathogenesis [24]. Compared to conventional immunosuppressive treatments, biologics modulate the inflammatory cascade with a high specificity by targeting a single molecule or receptor. Biologic agents include monoclonal antibodies and fusion proteins, which target proinflammatory cytokines or their receptors. Antibodies used as biologic drugs are either chimeric (mostly human-rodent) or completely humanized. Receptor constructs and immunomodulatory cytokines are also used as biologic agents [25–27].

How Safe Are Anti-Interleukin Agents?

Biologics have already been tested in large clinical trials for the treatment of rheumatoid arthritis (RA), psoriatic arthritis, and other forms of spondyloarthritis. Further experience comes from their use in Behçet's disease, chronic inflammatory bowel disease, or JIA. Uveitis can be associated with one of these diseases or present as isolated ocular inflammation.

In a large meta-analysis and Cochrane overview, Singh et al. [28] reviewed 163 randomized clinical trials with 50,010 patients and 46 extension studies with 11,954 patients for adverse effects. The safety profile for cytokine-inhibiting therapies, when used in approved indications such as RA, appears to be comparable to that of TNF-blocking agents. The increased risk of allergic reactions depends on the mode of application. Both minor and severe infections constitute typical side effects of any anti-cytokine therapy, but they are not observed any more frequently in IL blockade than in anti-TNF therapy. Some substance- or cytokine-specific side effects, e.g. on the metabolism during anti-IL-6 treatment, can be explained by the intrinsic function of the blocked mediator. An increased risk for lymphoma [29], which is already observed more frequently in RA and some other related disorders than in age-adjusted healthy populations, or other malignancies constitutes a general concern when using innovative therapies. Fortunately, no positive correlation between anti-IL treatment and malignancies has been reported from animal studies or from the limited clinical experience of IL inhibition, and even less has been reported concerning abortion or malformation rates in pregnancy. It is likely that any effect on pregnancy or an unborn child will differ from cytokine to cytokine. Indeed, most of the currently available recombinant proteins pass the placental barrier. Therefore, their use in pregnancy is subject to stringent restrictions.

Possible Indications for Anti-Interleukin Treatment

Decisions about uveitis treatment are based on the course of eye disease and also on the associated systemic disorder. Severity of ocular inflammation, the presence of sight-threatening complications, and response to previous treatments must be considered.

Mostly, a stepladder approach is used in the anti-inflammatory treatment of uveitis. The first choice is generally topical or systemic corticosteroid treatment (e.g. prednisolone 1 mg/kg body weight). For uveitis persisting with steroid dosages above the individual Cushing level, steroid-sparing agents are introduced, including anti-metabolites (azathioprine, methotrexate) and T cell inhibitors (cyclosporine A, mycophenolate mofetil). Inactivity cannot always be achieved, even by combining various immunosuppressives. In such instances, biologics offer a new therapeutic option. In addition to TNF-α inhibitors, several anti-IL drugs have been used to treat otherwise refractory uveitis. Unfortunately, no clinical trials have been conducted yet comparing the efficacy of the diverse biologics, given with or without combined immunosuppressives.

Interdisciplinary Approach in a Specialized Medical Care Unit

Due to their high costs and for safety reasons, anti-IL treatment is currently restricted to selected patients after a thorough interdisciplinary discussion among the treating uveitis specialist and experienced specialists from other disciplines. Although uveitis is less commonly associated with a systemic disease, it is essential that a rheumatologist be involved in the systemic workup and treatment discussion process. Prior to any biologic treatment, infectious diseases, malignancy, and certain immune-mediated entities must be excluded.

Anti-IL-1 Receptor Antagonist (Anakinra)

IL-1α and IL-1β are proinflammatory cytokines produced by many cells of the immune system, predominantly by activated macrophages, but also by B cells, cells of vascular endothelium, and other tissues. They were the first members of the growing family of IL-1-like proteins, including IL-18 and IL-33 [30].

In experimental animal models, increased levels of IL-1β can break down the blood-retinal barrier and attract polymorphonuclear cells and monocytes [31–34]. Furthermore, the importance of IL-1 has been shown for the Th17 cell generation and for the development of autoimmune responses [35]. IL-1R-deficient mice demonstrated less inflammation in an immune complex-induced uveitis model than did a control group [36]. In mice and rats, suppression of uveitis was achieved with IL-1R antagonists [37–40]. Increased levels of IL-1β have also been found in the serum or aqueous humor from patients with chronic uveitis [41, 42].

A review of 2,065 patients suffering from RA showed that anakinra, a recombinant IL-1 receptor antagonist, is modestly efficacious and relatively safe, although no long-term data are available yet [43]. The anti-IL-1R antibody anakinra is now approved for the treatment of RA in many countries. Furthermore, a meta-analysis of 140 children suffering from systemic JIA and treated with anakinra found a rapid response in otherwise therapy-resistant cases [44]. In contrast to anakinra treatment in RA, IL-1 blockade provides good to excellent efficacy in cryopyrin-associated familial syndromes (cold-associated fever, CINCA syndrome, and related diseases) and in crystal-induced forms of arthritis such as gout [45, 46]. Anakinra treatment must be administered daily; thus, IL-1-directed antibodies such as canakinumab with a longer half-life in the body were developed.

Regarding uveitis, the results of anakinra treatment have been encouraging in small groups of uveitis patients (e.g. for CINCA-associated uveitis, pars planitis, and ocular Behçet's disease) [47, 48].

Anti-IL-2 Receptor Antibody (Daclizumab)

IL-2 is a proinflammatory cytokine that is important for the induction and exacerbation of the effector response, for survival and for proliferation of T cells [49], and in activating B cells [50]. Therefore, IL-2 constitutes a potential target for an immunomodulatory treatment approach.

IL-2, which is expressed by activated Th1 effector cells, is one of the cytokines predominantly secreted in uveitis [23, 51]. Pato et al. [52] reviewed the efficacy of daclizumab, an anti-IL-2 receptor antibody, for the treatment of uveitis. In a randomized controlled trial, daclizumab was not effective in treating uveitis associated with Behçet's disease [53]. However, other case series revealed a possible effect of daclizumab for other forms of noninfectious uveitis and for the treatment of associated cystoid macular edema [54–57]. In a pilot study, Nussenblatt et al. [51] evaluated the value of daclizumab in treating sight-threatening, noninfectious intermediate uveitis, posterior uveitis, or panuveitis. In this prospective, multicenter, nonrandomized, noncomparative interventional trial, 10 of 15 patients achieved the primary end point of a ≥50% reduction of systemic corticosteroids and/or immunosuppressive regimens, and had maintained baseline visual acuity 12 and 26 weeks later. Furthermore, in other case series employing daclizumab for the treatment of birdshot chorioretinitis [58] or uveitis associated with JIA [59], inflammatory control was adequate in some patients refractory to other immunosuppressives.

In general, daclizumab was well tolerated. The reported adverse effects included nausea, fatigue, muscle aches, rashes, edema, upper respiratory infections, cutaneous herpes zoster lesions, hepatic dysfunction, or leukopenia. However, in 2009, the European Commission decided to withdraw authorization for daclizumab (Zenapax) after the responsible pharmaceutical company issued a voluntary request for commercial reasons.

Anti-IL-15 Antibody (HuMax-IL15)

The cytokine IL-15 is produced by mononuclear phagocytes [60]. Based on shared receptor components, IL-15 exacerbates some effects on cells of the innate and adaptive immune systems, similarly to IL-2 [61, 62]. IL-15 is an important factor for CD8+ memory T cell induction, maintenance and toxicity of NK cells, and activation, differentiation, and proliferation of B cells [63–66]. Furthermore, IL-15 can effectively inhibit TNF-α or FAS-L-mediated apoptosis [67, 68]. Together with IL-12, IL-15 induces IFN-γ and directs activated T cells towards a Th1 signature, which exerts several kinds of proinflammatory activity.

Elevated serum IL-15 levels have been found in patients with systemic autoimmune diseases, e.g. psoriasis, RA, ulcerative colitis, and Behçet's disease [69–71]. For RA, a clinical trial demonstrated significant improvement in disease activity without severe side effects for HuMax-IL15, a human monoclonal anti-IL-15 antibody [72]. Blocking IL-2 and IL-15 receptors reduced ocular inflammation in a monkey uveitis model [73]. However, up to now no clinical data are available concerning the use of an anti-IL-15 antibody to treat uveitis in humans.

Anti-IL-6 Receptor Antibody (Tocilizumab)

IL-6 is a pleiotropic cytokine that is mainly produced by T cells and monocytes/macrophages. It is a proinflammatory cytokine that induces proliferation and differentiation of T cells and terminal differentiation of B cells [74]. In the murine EAU model, IL-6 is a key player in generating Th17 cells, while it inhibits the generation of regulatory T cells [75, 76]. Thereby, IL-6 enhances acute inflammation and, furthermore, triggers the progression to chronic inflammation. Thus, in IL-6-deficient mice, the Th17 response was impaired and EAU scores were reduced [77]. In the liver, IL-6 is also essential for the induction of C-reactive protein and helps regulate anemia in chronic disease by inducing hepcidin, a mediator of ferroportin degradation and consequent blockade of iron uptake and iron retention in the reticuloendothelial system [78].

Increased serum levels of IL-6 have been found in various systemic autoimmune diseases, e.g. in RA, systemic lupus erythematosus, systemic-onset JIA, and Castleman's disease [79, 80]. Increased intraocular levels of IL-6 have been observed in idiopathic uveitis and in uveitis associated with Behçet's disease, sarcoidosis, Vogt-Koyanagi-Harada, ankylosing spondylitis, and Fuchs cyclitis [22].

Anti-IL-6R antibodies were effective in experimental models of autoimmune arthritis, encephalomyelitis, and also uveitis [77]. Tocilizumab, a fully humanized anti-IL-6R antibody, has been approved for the treatment of RA [74, 81]. Drug efficacy has also been shown in treating JIA [82–84] and vasculitis [85–87].

No clinical trials evaluating the use of an anti-IL-6R antibody in uveitis are available yet. We treated 3 adult patients with JIA-associated anterior uveitis in whom the condition was refractory to immunosuppressive agents (methotrexate or azathioprine) and anti-TNF-α inhibitors with tocilizumab infusions. With this treatment, uveitis inactivity was achieved in 2 of the 3 patients, and the associated arthritis improved in all of them [unpubl. obs.].

Anti-IL-17 Antibody (AIN457)

Th17 cells are specialized cells of the adaptive immune system which are involved in initiating an inflammatory response that is dominated by neutrophils [88]. Th17 cells contribute to several autoimmune diseases, e.g. multiple sclerosis [89] and RA [90]. These cells have also been found to be involved in the pathogenesis of uveitis in humans [91] and in a mouse model of EAU [92]. In mice with collagen-induced arthritis treated with anti-IL-17 antibodies, disease severity was significantly lower than in a control group [93]. In addition, the use of an anti-IL-17 antibody significantly reduced ocular inflammation in the murine model of EAU [92].

AIN457 is a fully humanized monoclonal antibody with a high affinity to IL-17A. This agent has proven efficacy in the treatment of psoriasis, RA, and uveitis [94]. Three placebo-controlled clinical trials to analyze the efficacy of AIN457 in intermediate, posterior, or panuveitis have been conducted: one for uveitis associated with Behçet's disease (SHIELD trial), a second one for quiescent uveitis (ENDURE trial), and the third for active uveitis (INSURE trial). The primary study outcome measure was defined as efficacy in maintaining/achieving the suppression of intraocular inflammation and reducing the ocular recurrence rate during withdrawal of concomitant immunosuppressive treatment. Secondary outcome measures included drug safety and improvement in visual acuity. The SHIELD trial for patients with uveitis associated with Behçet's disease did not meet the primary end point, as no statistically significant difference was found between AIN457 groups and the control group. The ENDURE and INSURE trials were also terminated ahead of time. Reasons for the termination are thought to be lack of efficacy after an interim analysis rather than safety issues.

Final Remarks

Further clinical trials including head-to-head comparative studies are required to define which specific drug should be favored in a distinct uveitis setting. Currently, biologic agents are not approved for treating uveitis, and therefore can only be administered as off-label agents. Due to the lack of clinical trials, health insurance companies are commonly reluctant to cover the expenses of the costly medication.

References

1 Rosenbaum JT, McDevitt HO, Guss RB, Egbert PR: Endotoxin-induced uveitis in rats as a model for human disease. Nature 1980;286:611–613.

2 Kogiso M, Tanouchi Y, Mimura Y, Nagasawa H, Himeno K: Endotoxin-induced uveitis in mice. 1. Induction of uveitis and role of T lymphocytes. Jpn J Ophthalmol 1992;36:281–290.

3 Bhattacherjee P, Williams RN, Eakins KE: An evaluation of ocular inflammation following the injection of bacterial endotoxin into the rat foot pad. Invest Ophthalmol Vis Sci 1983;24:196–202.

4 Forrester JV, Worgul BV, Merriam GR Jr: Endotoxin-induced uveitis in the rat. Graefes Arch Clin Exp Ophthalmol 1980;213:221–233.

5 Hoekzema R, Murray PI, van Haren MA, Helle M, Kijlstra A: Analysis of interleukin-6 in endotoxin-induced uveitis. Invest Ophthalmol Vis Sci 1991;32: 88–95.

6 Ohta K, Wiggert B, Yamagami S, Taylor AW, Streilein JW: Analysis of immunomodulatory activities of aqueous humor from eyes of mice with experimental autoimmune uveitis. J Immunol 2000; 164:1185–1192.

7 Xu Y, Chen W, Lu H, Hu X, Li S, Wang J, et al: The expression of cytokines in the aqueous humor and serum during endotoxin-induced uveitis in C3H/HeN mice. Mol Vis 2010;16:1689–1695.

8 Forrester JV, Liversidge J, Dua HS, Towler H, McMenamin PG: Comparison of clinical and experimental uveitis. Curr Eye Res 1990;9:75–84.

9 Atalla L, Linker-Israeli M, Steinman L, Rao NA: Inhibition of autoimmune uveitis by anti-CD4 antibody. Invest Ophthalmol Vis Sci 1990;31: 1264–1270.

10 Amadi-Obi A, Yu CR, Liu X, et al: T(H)17 cells contribute to uveitis and scleritis and are expanded by IL-2 and inhibited by IL-27/STAT1. Nature medicine 2007;13:711–718.

11 Rizzo LV, Silver P, Wiggert B, et al: Establishment and characterization of a murine CD4+ T cell line and clone that induce experimental autoimmune uveoretinitis in B10.A mice. J Immunol 1996;156: 1654–1660.

12 Caspi RR, Roberge FG, McAllister CG, El-Saied M, Kuwabara T, Gery I, et al: T cell lines mediating experimental autoimmune uveoretinitis (EAU) in the rat. J Immunol 1986;136:928–933.

13 Mochizuki M, Kuwabara T, McAllister C, Nussenblatt RB, Gery I: Adoptive transfer of experimental autoimmune uveoretinitis in rats. Immunopathogenic mechanisms and histologic features. Invest Ophthalmol Vis Sci 1985;26:1–9.

14 Caspi RR, Chan CC, Leake WC, Higuchi M, Wiggert B, Chader GJ: Experimental autoimmune uveoretinitis in mice. Induction by a single eliciting event and dependence on quantitative parameters of immunization. J Autoimmun 1990;3:237–246.

15 Caspi RR, Chan CC, Wiggert B, Chader GJ: The mouse as a model of experimental autoimmune uveoretinitis (EAU). Curr Eye Res 1990;9:169–174.

16 Chan CC, Caspi RR, Ni M, Leake WC, Wiggert B, Chader GJ, et al: Pathology of experimental autoimmune uveoretinitis in mice. J Autoimmun 1990;3: 247–255.
17 Xu H, Wawrousek EF, Redmond TM, Nickerson JM, Wiggert B, Chan CC, et al: Transgenic expression of an immunologically privileged retinal antigen extraocularly enhances self-tolerance and abrogates susceptibility to autoimmune uveitis. Eur J Immunol 2000;30:272–278.
18 Caspi RR: Understanding autoimmune uveitis through animal models. The Friedenwald Lecture. Invest Ophthalmol Vis Sci 2011;52:1872–1879.
19 Caspi RR: Immune mechanisms in uveitis. Springer Semin Immunopathol 1999;21:113–124.
20 Caspi R: Autoimmunity in the immune privileged eye: pathogenic and regulatory T cells. Immunol Res 2008;42:41–50.
21 Bettelli E, Korn T, Oukka M, Kuchroo VK: Induction and effector functions of T(H)17 cells. Nature 2008; 453:1051–1057.
22 Ooi KG-J, Galatowicz G, Calder VL, Lightman SL: Cytokines and chemokines in uveitis: is there a correlation with clinical phenotype? Clin Med Res 2006;4:294–309.
23 Caspi RR, Roberge FG, McAllister CG, el-Saied M, Kuwabara T, Gery I, et al: T cell lines mediating experimental autoimmune uveoretinitis (EAU) in the rat. J Immunol 1986;136:928–933.
24 Rosenbaum JT: Future for biological therapy for uveitis. Curr Opin Ophthalmol 2010;21:473–477.
25 Szekanecz Z, Szántó S, Szabó Z, Váncsa A, Szamosi S, Bodnár N, et al: Biologics – beyond the joints. Autoimmun Rev 2010;9:820–824.
26 Servat JJ, Mears KA, Black EH, Huang JJ: Biological agents for the treatment of uveitis. Expert Opin Biol Ther 2012, in press.
27 Imrie FR, Dick AD: Biologics in the treatment of uveitis. Curr Opin Ophthalmol 2007;18:481–486.
28 Singh JA, Wells GA, Christensen R, Tanjong Ghogomu E, Maxwell L, Macdonald JK, et al: Adverse effects of biologics: a network meta-analysis and Cochrane overview. Cochrane Database Syst Rev 2011;2:CD008794.
29 Baecklund E, Iliadou A, Askling J, Ekbom A, Backlin C, Granath F, et al: Association of chronic inflammation, not its treatment, with increased lymphoma risk in rheumatoid arthritis. Arthritis Rheum 2006; 54:692–701.
30 Gabay C, McInnes IB: The biological and clinical importance of the 'new generation' cytokines in rheumatic diseases. Arthritis Res Ther 2009;11:230.
31 Luna JD, Chan CC, Derevjanik NL, Mahlow J, Chiu C, Peng B, et al: Blood-retinal barrier (BRB) breakdown in experimental autoimmune uveoretinitis: comparison with vascular endothelial growth factor, tumor necrosis factor alpha, and interleukin-1beta-mediated breakdown. J Neurosci Res 1997;49: 268–280.
32 Claudio L, Martiney JA, Brosnan CF: Ultrastructural studies of the blood-retina barrier after exposure to interleukin-1 beta or tumor necrosis factor-alpha. Lab Invest 1994;70:850–861.
33 Ferrick MR, Thurau SR, Oppenheim MH, Herbort CP, Ni M, Zachariae CO, et al: Ocular inflammation stimulated by intravitreal interleukin-8 and interleukin-1. Invest Ophthalmol Vis Sci 1991;32: 1534–1539.
34 Bamforth SD, Lightman SL, Greenwood J: Interleukin-1 beta-induced disruption of the retinal vascular barrier of the central nervous system is mediated through leukocyte recruitment and histamine. Am J Pathol 1997;150:329–340.
35 Chung Y, Chang SH, Martinez GJ, Yang XO, Nurieva R, Kang HS, et al: Critical regulation of early Th17 cell differentiation by interleukin-1 signaling. Immunity 2009;30:576–587.
36 Brito BE, O'Rourke LM, Pan Y, Anglin J, Planck SR, Rosenbaum JT: IL-1 and TNF receptor-deficient mice show decreased inflammation in an immune complex model of uveitis. Invest Ophthalmol Vis Sci 1999;40:2583–2589.
37 Chiou GC, Xuan B, Liu Q, Yamasaki T, Okawara T: Inhibition of interleukin-1-induced uveitis and corneal fibroblast proliferation by interleukin-1 blockers. J Ocul Pharmacol Ther 2000;16:407–418.
38 Chiou GC, Chen Z, Xuan B, Yamasaki T, Okawara T: Antagonism of interleukin-1 (IL-1)-induced uveitis with synthetic IL-1 blockers. J Ocul Pharmacol Ther 1997;13:427–433.
39 Rosenbaum JT, Boney RS: Activity of an interleukin 1 receptor antagonist in rabbit models of uveitis. Arch Ophthalmol 1992;110:547–549.
40 Lim WK, Fujimoto C, Ursea R, Mahesh SP, Silver P, Chan CC, et al: Suppression of immune-mediated ocular inflammation in mice by interleukin 1 receptor antagonist administration. Arch Ophthalmol 2005;123:957–963.
41 Franks WA, Limb GA, Stanford MR, Ogilvie J, Wolstencroft RA, Chignell AH, et al: Cytokines in human intraocular inflammation. Curr Eye Res 1992;11:187–191.
42 El-Shabrawi YG, Christen WG, Foster SC: Correlation of metalloproteinase-2 and -9 with proinflammatory cytokines interleukin-1b, interleukin-12 and the interleukin-1 receptor antagonist in patients with chronic uveitis. Curr Eye Res 2000; 20:211–214.

43 Mertens M, Singh JA: Anakinra for rheumatoid arthritis: a systematic review. J Rheumatol 2009;36: 1118–1125.

44 Mertens M, Singh JA: Anakinra for rheumatoid arthritis. Cochrane Database Syst Rev 2009; CD005121.

45 So A, De Smedt T, Revaz S, Tschopp J: A pilot study of IL-1 inhibition by anakinra in acute gout. Arthritis Res Ther 2007;9:R28.

46 Busso N, So A: Mechanisms of inflammation in gout. Arthritis Res Ther 2010;12:206.

47 Teoh SCB, Sharma S, Hogan A, Lee R, Ramanan AV, Dick AD: Tailoring biological treatment: anakinra treatment of posterior uveitis associated with the CINCA syndrome. Br J Ophthalmol 2007;91: 263–264.

48 Benezra D, Maftzir G, Barak V: Blood serum interleukin-1 receptor antagonist in pars planitis and ocular Behçet disease. Am J Ophthalmol 1997;123: 593–598.

49 Gillis S, Mertelsmann R, Moore MA: T-cell growth factor (interleukin 2) control of T-lymphocyte proliferation: possible involvement in leukemogenesis. Transplant Proc 1981;13:1884–1890.

50 Zubler RH, Lowenthal JW, Erard F, Hashimoto N, Devos R, MacDonald HR: Activated B cells express receptors for, and proliferate in response to, pure interleukin 2. J Exp Med 1984;160:1170–1183.

51 Nussenblatt RB, Peterson JS, Foster CS, Rao NA, See RF, Letko E, et al: Initial evaluation of subcutaneous daclizumab treatments for noninfectious uveitis: a multicenter noncomparative interventional case series. Ophthalmology 2005;112:764–770.

52 Pato E, Muñoz-Fernández S, Francisco F, Abad MA, Maese J, Ortiz A, et al: Systematic review on the effectiveness of immunosuppressants and biological therapies in the treatment of autoimmune posterior uveitis. Semin Arthritis Rheum 2011;40:314–323.

53 Buggage RR, Levy-Clarke G, Sen HN, Ursea R, Srivastava SK, Suhler EB, et al: A double-masked, randomized study to investigate the safety and efficacy of daclizumab to treat the ocular complications related to Behçet's disease. Ocul Immunol Inflamm 2007;15:63–70.

54 Gallagher M, Quinones K, Cervantes-Castañeda RA, Yilmaz T, Foster CS: Biological response modifier therapy for refractory childhood uveitis. Br J Ophthalmol 2007;91:1341–1344.

55 Papaliodis GN, Chu D, Foster CS: Treatment of ocular inflammatory disorders with daclizumab. Ophthalmology 2003;110:786–789.

56 Hernández Garfella ML, Díaz-Llopis M, Salom Alonso D, Cervera Taulet E: Recurrent uveitis and therapy with monoclonal antibody (daclizumab) (in Spanish). Arch Soc Esp Oftalmol 2004;79:593–598.

57 Nussenblatt RB, Fortin E, Schiffman R, Rizzo L, Smith J, van Veldhuisen P, et al: Treatment of noninfectious intermediate and posterior uveitis with the humanized anti-Tac mAb: a phase I/II clinical trial. Proc Natl Acad Sci USA 1999;96:7462–7466.

58 Sobrin L, Huang JJ, Christen W, Kafkala C, Choopong P, Foster CS: Daclizumab for treatment of birdshot chorioretinopathy. Arch Ophthalmol 2008;126:186–191.

59 Sen HN, Levy-Clarke G, Faia LJ, Li Z, Yeh S, Barron KS, et al: High-dose daclizumab for the treatment of juvenile idiopathic arthritis-associated active anterior uveitis. Am J Ophthalmol 2009;148:696–703.e1.

60 Doherty TM, Seder RA, Sher A: Induction and regulation of IL-15 expression in murine macrophages. J Immunol 1996;156:735–741.

61 Giri JG, Ahdieh M, Eisenman J, Shanebeck K, Grabstein K, Kumaki S, et al: Utilization of the beta and gamma chains of the IL-2 receptor by the novel cytokine IL-15. EMBO J 1994;13:2822–2830.

62 Giri JG, Anderson DM, Kumaki S, Park LS, Grabstein KH, Cosman D: IL-15, a novel T cell growth factor that shares activities and receptor components with IL-2. J Leukoc Biol 1995;57: 763–766.

63 Armitage RJ, Macduff BM, Eisenman J, Paxton R, Grabstein KH: IL-15 has stimulatory activity for the induction of B cell proliferation and differentiation. J Immunol 1995;154:483–490.

64 Carson WE, Giri JG, Lindemann MJ, Linett ML, Ahdieh M, Paxton R, et al: Interleukin (IL) 15 is a novel cytokine that activates human natural killer cells via components of the IL-2 receptor. J Exp Med 1994;180:1395–1403.

65 Dunne J, Lynch S, O'Farrelly C, Todryk S, Hegarty JE, Feighery C, et al: Selective expansion and partial activation of human NK cells and NK receptor-positive T cells by IL-2 and IL-15. J Immunol 2001;167: 3129–3138.

66 Hébert P, Pruett SB: Selective loss of viability of mouse NK cells in culture is associated with decreased NK cell lytic function. In Vitr Mol Toxicol 2001;14:71–82.

67 Bulfone-PauS S, Bulanova E, Bulfone-Paus E, Pohl T, Budagian V, Durkop H, et al: Death deflected: IL-15 inhibits TNF-alpha-mediated apoptosis in fibroblasts by TRAF2 recruitment to the IL-15Ralpha chain. FASEB J 1999;13:1575–1585.

68 Bulfone-PauS S, Ungureanu D, Pohl T, Lindner G, Paus R, Ruckert R, et al: Interleukin-15 protects from lethal apoptosis in vivo. Nat Med 1997;3: 1124–1128.

69 McInnes IB, Gracie JA: Interleukin-15: a new cytokine target for the treatment of inflammatory diseases. Curr Opin Pharmacol 2004;4:392–397.

70 Kirman I, Vainer B, Nielsen OH: Interleukin-15 and its role in chronic inflammatory diseases. Inflamm Res 1998;47:285–289.
71 Hamzaoui K, Hamzaoui A, Ghorbel I, Khanfir M, Houman H: Levels of IL-15 in serum and cerebrospinal fluid of patients with Behçet's disease. Scand J Immunol 2006;64:655–660.
72 Baslund B, Tvede N, Danneskiold-Samsoe B, Larsson P, Panayi G, Petersen J, et al: Targeting interleukin-15 in patients with rheumatoid arthritis: a proof-of-concept study. Arthritis Rheum 2005; 52:2686–2692.
73 Guex-Crosier Y, Raber J, Chan CC, Kriete MS, Benichou J, Pilson RS, et al: Humanized antibodies against the alpha-chain of the IL-2 receptor and against the beta-chain shared by the IL-2 and IL-15 receptors in a monkey uveitis model of autoimmune diseases. J Immunol 1997;158:452–458.
74 Mima T, Nishimoto N: Clinical value of blocking IL-6 receptor. Curr Opin Rheumatol 2009;21: 224–230.
75 Bettelli E, Carrier Y, Gao W, Korn T, Strom TB, Oukka M, et al: Reciprocal developmental pathways for the generation of pathogenic effector TH17 and regulatory T cells. Nature 2006;441:235–238.
76 Korn T, Mitsdoerffer M, Croxford AL, Awasthi A, Dardalhon VA, Galileos G, et al: IL-6 controls Th17 immunity in vivo by inhibiting the conversion of conventional T cells into Foxp3+ regulatory T cells. Proc Natl Acad Sci USA 2008;105:18460–18465.
77 Yoshimura T, Sonoda K-H, Ohguro N, Ohsugi Y, Ishibashi T, Cua DJ, et al: Involvement of Th17 cells and the effect of anti-IL-6 therapy in autoimmune uveitis. Rheumatology (Oxford) 2009;48:347–354.
78 Weiss G, Goodnough LT: Anemia of chronic disease. N Engl J Med 2005;352:1011–1023.
79 Nishimoto N, Kishimoto T: Interleukin 6: from bench to bedside. Nat Clin Pract Rheumatol 2006; 2:619–626.
80 Ishihara K, Hirano T: IL-6 in autoimmune disease and chronic inflammatory proliferative disease. Cytokine Growth Factor Rev 2002;13:357–368.
81 Ohsugi Y, Kishimoto T: The recombinant humanized anti-IL-6 receptor antibody tocilizumab, an innovative drug for the treatment of rheumatoid arthritis. Expert Opin Biol Ther 2008;8:669–681.
82 Mircic M, Kavanaugh A: Inhibition of IL6 in rheumatoid arthritis and juvenile idiopathic arthritis. Exp Cell Res 2011;317:1286–1292.
83 Yokota S, Kishimoto T: Tocilizumab: molecular intervention therapy in children with systemic juvenile idiopathic arthritis. Expert Rev Clin Immunol 2010;6:735–743.
84 Herlin T: Tocilizumab: The evidence for its place in the treatment of juvenile idiopathic arthritis. Core Evid 2010;4:181–189.
85 Seitz M, Reichenbach S, Bonel HM, Adler S, Wermelinger F, Villiger PM: Rapid induction of remission in large vessel vasculitis by IL-6 blockade. A case series. Swiss Med Wkly 2011;141:w13156.
86 Nishimoto N, Nakahara H, Yoshio-Hoshino N, Mima T: Successful treatment of a patient with Takayasu arteritis using a humanized anti-interleukin-6 receptor antibody. Arthritis Rheum 2008;58: 1197–1200.
87 Borhani Haghighi A, Safari A: Tocilizumab may be a potential addition to our weapons against neuro-Behçet's disease. Med Hypotheses 2008;71:156–157.
88 Zhang Z, Zhong W, Spencer D, Chen H, Lu H, Kawaguchi T, et al: Interleukin-17 causes neutrophil mediated inflammation in ovalbumin-induced uveitis in DO11.10 mice. Cytokine 2009;46:79–91.
89 Tzartos JS, Friese MA, Craner MJ, Palace J, Newcombe J, Esiri MM, et al: Interleukin-17 production in central nervous system-infiltrating T cells and glial cells is associated with active disease in multiple sclerosis. Am J Pathol 2008;172:146–155.
90 Shahrara S, Huang Q, Mandelin AM, Pope RM: TH-17 cells in rheumatoid arthritis. Arthritis Res Ther 2008;10:R93.
91 Chi W, Zhu X, Yang P, Liu X, Lin X, Zhou H, et al: Upregulated IL-23 and IL-17 in Behçet patients with active uveitis. Invest Ophthalmol Vis Sci 2008;49: 3058–3064.
92 Amadi-Obi A, Yu C-R, Liu X, Mahdi RM, Clarke GL, Nussenblatt RB, et al: TH17 cells contribute to uveitis and scleritis and are expanded by IL-2 and inhibited by IL-27/STAT1. Nat Med 2007;13:711–718.
93 Lubberts E, Koenders MI, Oppers-Walgreen B, van den Bersselaar L, Coenen-de Roo CJJ, Joosten LAB, et al: Treatment with a neutralizing anti-murine interleukin-17 antibody after the onset of collagen-induced arthritis reduces joint inflammation, cartilage destruction, and bone erosion. Arthritis Rheum 2004;50:650–659.
94 Hueber W, Patel DD, Dryja T, Wright AM, Koroleva I, Bruin G, et al: Effects of AIN457, a fully human antibody to interleukin-17A, on psoriasis, rheumatoid arthritis, and uveitis. Sci Transl Med 2010;2: 52ra72.

Christoph Tappeiner, MD, FEBO
Department of Ophthalmology, Inselspital, University of Bern
CH–3010 Bern (Switzerland)
Tel. +41 31 632 85 03, E-Mail christoph.tappeiner@insel.ch

Miserocchi E, Modorati G, Foster CS (eds): New Treatments in Noninfectious Uveitis.
Dev Ophthalmol. Basel, Karger, 2012, vol 51, pp 90–97

Interferon-α Therapy in Noninfectious Uveitis

Christoph Deuter[a] · Nicole Stübiger[b] · Manfred Zierhut[a]

[a]Centre for Ophthalmology, University of Tübingen, Tübingen, and [b]Department of Ophthalmology, Campus Benjamin Franklin, Charité, Universitätsmedizin Berlin, Berlin, Germany

Abstract

Interferon (IFN)-α and IFN-β are naturally occurring cytokines which seem to have similar effects on the immune system. One of the effects of IFN seems to increase regulatory T cells. There are numerous case reports and studies reporting about the effect of IFN-α against Behçet's disease (BD), but also against chronic uveitic macular edema and a few other types of uveitis. Within 2–4 weeks, approximately 94% of patients reach complete or partial remission in the case of BD-associated uveitis. So far, IFN-α is the only drug that leads to stable remission even after discontinuation of the treatment. It is recommended to start treatment with 3–6 million IU per day. Administering less than daily dosages seems to increase the recurrence rate for BD-associated uveitis. Flu-like symptoms are expected in all patients as a sign of nonexisting anti-IFN antibodies. They are treated with nonsteroidal anti-inflammatory drugs like paracetamol and disappear normally after some days. Depression (8%) and mild leukopenia (30%) are additional side effects of concern; all other side effects are reported to appear in ≤1% of cases. This chapter updates the mechanisms and pharmacology of IFN and its effects in experimental studies. This is followed by a summary of clinical studies in intraocular inflammation and the spectrum of side effects.

Interferon (IFN)-α and IFN-β, which belong to the type I IFNs, are naturally occurring cytokines. There is about 30% homology of amino acid sequence. Both IFNs are sharing the same receptor; therefore, the therapeutic effect of these IFNs seems to be quite similar. Besides being approved as single agents for the treatment of adults with chronic hepatitis B and C, various hematologic malignancies, malignant melanoma and multiple sclerosis [1–4], there is growing evidence that especially IFN-α is highly effective in the treatment of Behçet's disease (BD) and also chronic uveitic macular edema.

Mechanisms and Pharmacology

IFN-α is a naturally occurring cytokine and belongs, same as IFN-β, to the type I IFNs. In general, any cell can produce type I IFNs, but antigen-presenting cells,

Table 1. Overview regarding the commercially available IFN-α and IFN-β

Trade name	Pharmaceutical company	Agent
Roferon A®	Hoffmann LaRoche	IFN-α2a
Pegasys®	Hoffmann LaRoche	pegylated IFN-α2a
Intron A®	Essex Pharma	IFN-α2b
PegIntron®	Essex Pharma	pegylated IFN-α2b
Avonex®	Biogen	IFN-β1a
Rebif®	Merck Serono	IFN-β1a
Betaferon®	Bayer Schering Pharma	IFN-β1b
Extavia®	Novartis	IFN-β1b

especially plasmacytoid dendritic cells, are the main producers of type I IFNs, already at early stages of the immune response. Thus, type I IFNs, especially IFN-α, may be the essential cytokines linking the innate with the adaptive immune system. Low levels of type I IFNs seem to be preconditions for the upregulation of type I IFNs as a reaction to viral infection and subsequent induction of IFN-γ production. This finally leads to the induction and maintenance of T helper type 1 cells, CD8+ cytotoxic T cells, and natural killer cells. In contrast, type I IFNs have also been shown to exert an antiproliferative and an apoptotic effect on T cells. Another IFN effect is the development of tolerance-promoting regulatory T cells. There has been a positive as well as an inhibitory effect described on B cell development and survival [5, 6].

Using in vitro studies, Plskova et al. [7] had found that plasmacytoid dendritic cells of patients with posterior uveitis induce less IFN-α after stimulation than cells from healthy controls. In addition, TNF-α was able to reduce the IFN-α levels by inhibition of number and function of IFN-α-generating dendritic cells [8].

It has been shown that numbers of γ-δ T cells were normalized [9] and soluble TNF receptors increased in BD patients treated with IFN [10]. Regulatory T cells also seem to play a key role in the effect of IFN. Therefore, a significant increase in Foxp3 expression of regulatory T cells (CD4+CD25^{high}) has been demonstrated for patients with BD treated for 6 months with IFN-α, and also for patients with multiple sclerosis treated for 12 months with IFN-β [11, 12]. This effect was not detectable in BD patients treated with immunosuppression.

IFN-α was the first cytokine to be produced in the recombinant form in the early 1980s. Nowadays, different types of human recombinant IFN-α and IFN-β (table 1) given subcutaneously are available. In general, the original formulation requires daily injections, but the development of pegylated versions, with the addition of polyethylene glycol to the standard structure, allows for much lower doses and convenient application only once a week. The pegylation results in a biologically active molecule with more sustained absorption and a longer half-life [13].

During tubular reabsorption, IFN undergoes proteolytic degradation, and it is completely filtered in the kidneys. Depending on the mode of application (subcutaneously, intramuscularly, or intravenously), the mean half-life of the standard IFNs is 2–5 h [14]. IFN is not considered to be safe in pregnancy [14].

Experimental Work

Today, there is only limited information about the effect of IFN in experimental uveitis work. In 1998, Okada et al. [15] used the IRBP model to show suppression of inflammation in IFN type I-treated rats, suggesting that this suppression may be mediated in part by a reduction in TNF-α [15]. This group [16] found the same effect based on an increased production of NK cells and NKT cells. Recently, it has been shown that subretinal delivery of AAV2.hIFN-α can lead to an effective expression within the eye for at least 3 months, and that it significantly attenuates experimental autoimmune uveoretinitis activity [17].

Clinical Effects

Today, the most common indication for IFN-α in ophthalmology is ocular involvement due to BD. BD is a systemic immune-mediated vasculitis of unclear origin. Major symptoms include oral aphthous ulcers, genital ulcerations, skin manifestations, and intraocular inflammation. The latter is characterized by a recurrent posterior or panuveitis and by an occlusive retinal vasculitis that is responsible for the poor visual prognosis of this uveitis entity [18]. It is estimated that without treatment more than 90% of patients become blind after less than 4 years of disease [19]. Since the mid-1980s, a rising number of case series and open studies reported about the favorable effect of IFN-α in the treatment of BD, and especially of acute episodes of severe uveitis. A review of the literature by Kötter et al. [20] analyzing 32 original reports and 4 selected abstracts revealed that between 1986 and 2002 a total of 338 BD patients have been treated with IFN-α; in 182 of them acute uveitis was the indication. Within 2–4 weeks, approximately 94% of patients achieved complete or partial remission of ocular disease. The data of a prospective open study conducted by our group showed that IFN-α works fast enough to be suitable as a rescue therapy for acute relapses of BD uveitis. The study included 50 patients with active sight-threatening panuveitis and/or retinal vasculitis unresponsive to at least one immunosuppressive drug. Treatment efficacy was assessed using the 'uveitis scoring system' by BenEzra et al. [21]. More than 90% of patients responded to treatment and achieved complete remission of ocular disease within a median of 4 weeks. Mean posterior uveitis score fell by 46% per week. Cystoid macular edema (CME), if present, disappeared in all eyes [22]. Similar results have been published by Tugal-Tutkun et al. [23]. In a

Table 2. Long-term data for IFN-α in ocular BD from different studies

	Krause et al. [27]	Gueudry et al. [26]	Deuter et al. [28]
Patients	45	32	53
Follow-up, years	6.67 (0.3–22.3)	5.53 (1.3–10.8)	6.0 (2.0–12.6)
Responders	39 (87%)	28 (87.5%)	52 (98.1%)
Patients who were able to discontinue IFN-α in remission	9 (20%)	19 (68%)	47 (88.7%)
Mean treatment duration, months	33	32	22.4
Relapse-free patients	9 (20%)	13 (68%)	27 (57.4%)
Mean relapse-free period, months	37 (2–113)	43 (11–84)	45.9
Eyes with stable or improved visual acuity	91%	87.5%	94.8%

retrospective study on 44 BD patients with unresponsive BD uveitis, 91% of patients showed complete or partial response. A significant improvement in visual acuity also occurred. However, the authors postulated possible differences in therapeutic efficacy and side effect profile of IFN-α in different patient populations. Under treatment with IFN-α, the reperfusion of occluded retinal vessels as well as a complete regression of retinal neovascularization have been reported [24, 25]. Thus, we found that, if IFN-α is used in time, retinal laser photocoagulation can be avoided in almost all patients with ocular BD.

A major problem in the treatment of BD uveitis is the fact that despite early use of immunosuppressive drugs like cyclosporine or azathioprine, a substantial proportion of patients will lose useful vision over time. Thus, we have to redefine the goal in the treatment of BD uveitis which today has to be preservation of good visual function by avoiding relapses. Recently, three studies with a total of 130 patients [26–28] demonstrated that this goal can be achieved with the use of IFN-α (table 2). So far, this cytokine is the only drug that allows patients with BD uveitis to stay in remission even after complete discontinuation of treatment. As a consequence of the favorable therapeutic effects, IFN-α has been included in the EULAR recommendation for treatment of BD equal to TNF-blocking agents [29].

Despite the long-standing experience with IFN-α in BD, uniform dosing regimens still do not exist. An analysis of the literature suggests that intermediate to high doses are more effective and long-term remission seems to be associated with higher doses of IFN-α but not with longer treatment durations [20]. Therefore, we tend to start IFN-α treatment with high initial doses such as 3–6 million IU per day, depending on the body weight of the patients. We also highly recommend to stop other immunosuppressive drugs completely on the day before start of IFN-α and to taper systemic corticosteroids

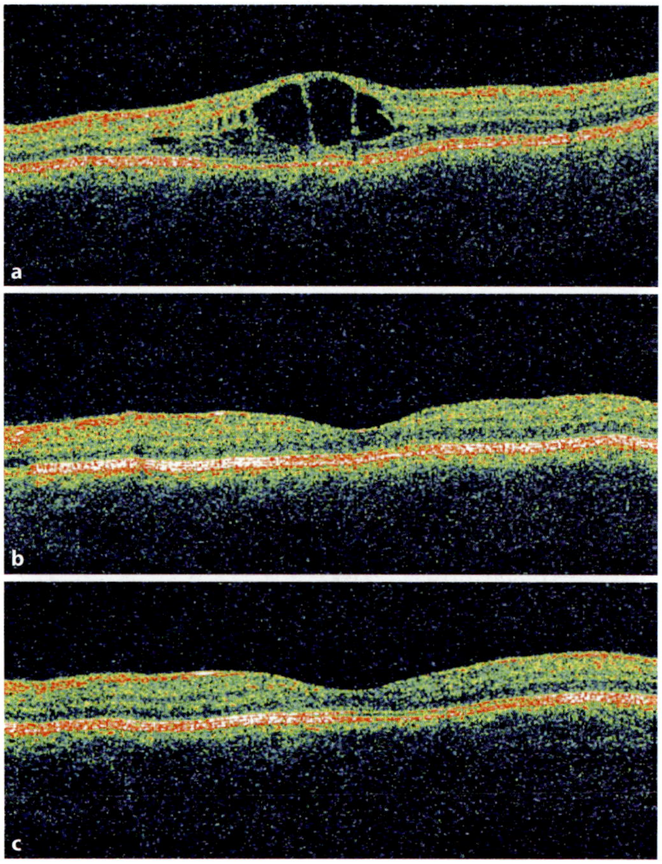

Fig. 1. A 32-year-old female with unresponsive CME since 17 months due to noninfectious intermediate uveitis (left eye). Ineffective pretreatment included systemic prednisolone, acetazolamide, mycophenolate mofetil, voclosporin, and intravitreal bevacizumab. **a** Optical coherence tomography (OCT) before initiation of IFN-α. CME with central foveal thickness (CFT) of 570 μm, visual acuity (VA) = 20/40. **b** OCT after 2 weeks on IFN-α shows almost complete resolution of CME. CFT = 190 μm; VA = 20/20. **c** OCT after 3 months on IFN-α. No CME is visible. CFT = 180 μm; VA = 20/25.

to a dose of 10 mg prednisolone equivalent per day as soon as possible because it has been postulated that these drugs may antagonize the therapeutic effect of IFN-α [18].

Based on the observation that the use of IFN-α alone (without other drugs like corticosteroids, acetazolamide and immunosuppressives) leads to complete regression of CME in ocular BD, the idea came up to use this drug also for chronic CME due to noninfectious non-BD uveitis. Although we have to assume meanwhile that the mode of action is probably different in both entities, the treatment of chronic uveitic CME with IFN-α passed through a very promising development. In 2009, we reported on 24 patients that we have treated with IFN-α for chronic long-standing uveitic CME unresponsive to systemic or local corticosteroids, acetazolamide and immunosuppressives. Within 3 months, IFN-α led to complete or partial resorption of CME in 87.5% of patients. It was impressive how fast IFN-α works in this indication. So, in most patients a response of CME was already seen after 3 days (fig. 1). However, in contrast to ocular BD, the vast majority of patients with chronic uveitic CME is not able to discontinue IFN-α but needs a long-term treatment at very low maintenance doses to keep absence of CME [30]. To date, we started IFN-α in 58 patients of whom 38 completed a follow-up of at least 24 months. Of the latter, 74% were still on IFN-α treatment after a mean follow-up of 56 months [Deuter et al., unpubl. data]. Meanwhile, our experiences have been confirmed by a group from France that treated 6 patients with chronic uveitic CME. All of them responded to treatment with IFN-α [31]. As aggressive anti-inflammatory treatment with immunosuppressive or even TNF-blocking agents does not work in chronic uveitic CME but IFN-α does, the mode of action of IFN-α cannot or cannot only be anti-inflammatory in this indication. Fitting with this hypothesis, in vitro experiments showed that IFN-α improves the endothelial barrier function of small retinal vessels [32]. Interestingly, IFN-α shows also promising effects in another form of chronic CME with an inflammatory background that is Irvine-Gass syndrome [33], but in our experience it is less or not effective in other (not primary inflammatory) types of CME (e.g. due to diabetes, central vein occlusion, retinitis pigmentosa). In contrast to ocular BD, previous immunosuppressive treatment does not have to be discontinued when IFN-α is given for chronic uveitic CME.

One of the most devastating forms of intraocular inflammation is serpiginous choroiditis. One case series reports on the successful use of IFN-α in this indication. Sobaci et al. [34] treated 5 patients with active sight-threatening serpiginous choroiditis that was refractory to conventional immunosuppressive treatment, with IFN-α. All active lesions resolved within 6 months, recurrences could be prevented, useful vision recovered or maintained during a follow-up of 16–48 months.

Side Effects

Ninety percent of the patients suffer from flu-like symptoms, which mostly resolve during the first weeks after initiation of IFN. Application of nonsteroidal anti-inflammatory drugs (e.g. paracetamol) can often ease this problem. However, the development of these symptoms is a good marker that the IFN therapy is effective. The absence of flu-like symptoms seems to be an indicator for preexisting (or newly formed) anti-IFN autoantibodies [20, 30, 35]. Other adverse side effects are reddening at the side of injection, mild leukopenia (30%), alopecia (10%), depression (8%), gastrointestinal disturbances (>1%), increase in liver enzymes (<1%), transient paresthesias (<1%) and other central nervous system symptoms, e.g. epilepsy (<1%) [7, 20, 22, 35]. Another severe adverse event is the development of anti-DNA and anti-thyroid antibodies (less than 1% of treated patients), which can rarely cause exacerbation or new onset of autoimmune disease [20, 22, 36].

Apart from that, the occurrence of sarcoidosis and Vogt-Koyanagi-Harada syndrome has been observed during therapy with IFN-α [13, 37]. Interestingly, the known development of an IFN retinopathy in hepatitis patients and in patients with posterior uveitis, which is not BD associated, was never found in patients with ocular BD [7, 20, 22].

In general, 4–7.5% of patients experienced side effects during IFN therapy, which were severe enough to warrant discontinuation [22, 25, 35].

Conclusion

The use of IFN-α has strongly improved the prognosis of BD. It seems to be the only drug available which can be stopped and still lead to lasting remission. There is no general agreement about the dosage, but it seems that starting with dosages less than daily may lead to a higher recurrence rate. In addition, IFN-α also has shown to be very effective for the treatment of chronic uveitic macular edema. In contrast to BD uveitis, most of the patients require a minimal basic dosage for continuing a dry macula. How IFN reduces the inflammation and also the edema of the macula is unclear at this moment, but the effectiveness has been shown in various studies.

References

1 Stoutenburg JP, Schrope B, Kaufmann HL: Adjuvant therapy for malignant melanoma. Expert Rev Anticancer Ther 2004;8:823–835.

2 Saadeh S, Davis GL: The evolving treatment of chronic hepatitis C: where we stand a decade out. Cleve Clin J Med 2004;71:3–7.

3 Okada H, Pollack IF: Cytokine gene therapy for malignant glioma. Expert Opin Biol Ther 2004;4: 1609–1620.

4 Green AR, Vassilou GS, Curtin N, Campbell PJ: Management of the myeloproliferative disorders: distinguishing data from dogma. Hematol J 2004;5: 126–132.

5 Theofilopoulos AN, Baccala R, Beutler B, Kono DH: Type I interferons (alpha/beta) in immunity and autoimmunity. Annu Rev Immunol 2005;23: 307–336.

6 Baccala R, Hoebe K, Kono DH, Beutler B, Theofilopoulos AN: TLR-dependent and TLR-independent pathways of type I interferon induction in systemic autoimmunity. Nat Med 2007;13: 543–551.

7 Plskova J, Greiner K, Forrester JV: Interferon-α as an effective treatment for noninfectious posterior uveitis and panuveitis. Am J Ophthalmol 2007;144: 55–61.

8 Plskova J, Greiner K, Muckersie, et al: Interferon-alpha: a key factor in autoimmune disease? Invest Ophthalmol Vis Sci 2006:47:3946–3950.

9 Treusch M, Vonthein R, Baur M, Günaydin I, Koch S, Stübiger N, Eckstein AK, Peter HH, Ness T, Zierhut M, Kötter I: Influence of human recombinant interferon-alpha2a (rhIFN-alpha2a) on altered lymphocyte subpopulations and monocytes in Behcet's disease. Rheumatology (Oxford) 2004;43: 1275–1282.

10 Kötter I, Deuter C, Stübiger N, Zierhut M: Interferon-α (IFN-α) application versus tumor necrosis factor-α antagonism for ocular Behcet's disease: focusing more on IFN. J Rheumatol 2005; 32:1633, author reply 1634.

11 Vandenbark AA, Huan J, Agotsch M, et al: Interferon-beta-1a treatment increases CD56 (bright) natural killer cells and CD4+CD25+Foxp3 expression in subjects with multiple sclerosis. J Neuroimmunol 2009;215:125–128.

12 Yang DS, Galatowicz G, Calder VL: Upregulation of Foxp3 expression by recombinant interferon-alpha therapy in Behcet's disease; in ARVO, Fort Lauderdale, 2009; poster 1535.

13 Hurst EA, Mauro T: Sarcoidosis associated with pegylated interferon alfa and ribavirin treatment for chronic hepatitis C: a case report and review of the literature. Arch Dermatol 2005;141:865–868.

14 Okada AA: Immunomodulatory therapy for ocular inflammatory disease: a basic manual and review of the literature. Ocul Immunol Inflamm 2005;13: 335–351.

15 Okada AA, Keino H, Fukai T, et al: Effect of type I interferon on experimental autoimmune uveoretinitis in rats. Ocul Immunol Inflamm 1998;6:209–210.

16 Suzuki J, Sakai J, Okada AA: Oral administration of interferon-alpha suppresses experimental autoimmune uveoretinitis. Graefes Archiv Clin Exp Ophthalmol 2002;240:314–321.
17 Tian L, Yang P, Lei B, Shao J, Wang C, Xiang Q, Wei L, Peng Z, Kijlstra A: AAV2-mediated subretinal gene transfer of hIFN-alpha attenuates experimental autoimmune uveoretinitis in mice. PLoS One 2011;6:e19542.
18 Deuter CME, Kötter I, Wallace GR, Murray PI, Stübiger N, Zierhut M: Behçet's disease: ocular effects and treatment. Prog Ret Eye Res 2008;27:111–136.
19 Mamo JG: The rate of visual loss in Behçet's disease. Arch Ophthalmol 1970;84:451–452.
20 Kötter I, Günaydin I, Zierhut M, Stübiger N: The use of interferon α in Behçet disease: review of the literature. Semin Arthritis Rheum 2004;33:320–355.
21 BenEzra D, Forrester JV, Nussenblatt RB, Tabbara K, Timonen P: Uveitis Scoring System. Berlin, Springer, 1991.
22 Kötter I, Zierhut M, Eckstein AK, Vonthein R, Ness T, Günaydin I, Grimbacher B, Blaschke S, Meyer-Riemann W, Peter HH, Stübiger N: Human recombinant interferon alfa-2a for the treatment of Behçet's disease with sight threatening posterior or panuveitis. Br J Ophthalmol 2003;87:423–431.
23 Tugal-Tutkun I, Güney-Tefekli E, Urgancioglu M: Results of interferon-alfa therapy in patients with Behçet uveitis. Graefes Arch Clin Exp Ophthalmol 2006;244:1692–1695.
24 Stübiger N, Kötter I, Zierhut M: Complete regression of retinal neovascularisation after therapy with interferon alfa in Behçet's disease. Br J Ophthalmol 2000;84:1437–1438.
25 Tugal-Tutkun I, Onal S, Altan-Yaycioglu R, Kir N, Urgancioglu M: Neovascularization of the optic disc in Behçet's disease. Jpn J Ophthalmol 2006;50: 256–265.
26 Gueudry J, Wechsler B, Terrada C, Gendron G, Cassoux N, Fardeau C, LeHoang P, Piette JC, Bodaghi B: Long-term efficacy and safety of low-dose interferon alpha2a therapy in severe uveitis associated with Behçet disease. Am J Ophthalmol 2008;146:837–844.
27 Krause L, Altenburg A, Pleyer U, Köhler AK, Zouboulis CC, Förster MH: Longterm visual prognosis of patients with ocular Adamantiades-Behçet's disease treated with interferon-α-2a. J Rheumatol 2008;35:896–903.
28 Deuter CME, Zierhut M, Möhle A, Vonthein R, Stübiger N, Kötter I: Long-term remission after cessation of interferon-α treatment in patients with severe uveitis due to Behçet's disease. Arthritis Rheum 2010;62:2796–2805.
29 Hatemi G, Silman A, Bang D, Bodaghi B, Chamberlain AM, Gul A, Houman MH, Kötter I, Olivieri I, Salvarani C, Sfikakis PP, Siva A, Stanford MR, Stübiger N, Yurdakul S, Yazici H, EULAR Expert Committee: EULAR recommendations for the management of Behçet disease. Ann Rheum Dis 2008;67:1656–1662.
30 Deuter CM, Kötter I, Günaydin I, Stübiger N, Doycheva DG, Zierhut M: Efficacy and tolerability of interferon alpha treatment in patients with chronic cystoid macular oedema due to non-infectious uveitis. Br J Ophthalmol 2009;93: 906–913.
31 Paire V, Lebreton O, Weber M: Effectiveness of interferon alpha in the treatment of uveitis macular edema refractory to corticosteroid and/or immunosuppressive treatment. J Fr Ophthalmol 2010;33: 152–162.
32 Gillies MC, Su T: Interferon-alpha 2b enhances barrier function of bovine retinal microvascular endothelium in vitro. Microvasc Res 1995;49:277–288.
33 Deuter CME, Gelisken F, Stübiger N, Zierhut M, Doycheva D: Successful treatment of chronic pseudophakic macular edema (Irvine-Gass syndrome) with interferon alpha: a report of three cases. Ocul Immunol Inflamm 2011;19:216–218.
34 Sobaci G, Bayraktar Z, Bayer A: Interferon alpha-2a treatment for serpiginous choroiditis. Ocul Immunol Inflamm 2005;13:59–66.
35 Bodaghi B, Gendron G, Wechsler B, et al: Efficacy of interferon alpha in the treatment of refractory and sight threatening uveitis: a retrospective monocentric study of 45 patients. Br J Ophthalmol 2007;91:35–339.
36 Conlon KC, Urba WJ, Smith JW, et al: Exacerbation of symptoms of autoimmune disease in patients receiving interferon-alpha therapy. Cancer 1990;65: 2237–2242.
37 Doycheva D, Deuter CME, Stübiger N et al: Interferon-alpha associated presumed ocular sarcoidosis. Graefes Arch Clin Exp Ophthalmol 2009; 247:675–680.

Manfred Zierhut
Centre for Ophthalmology, University of Tübingen
Schleichstrasse 12–16
DE–72076 Tübingen (Germany)
Tel. +49 7071 298 4008, E-Mail manfred.zierhut@med.uni-tuebingen.de

Miserocchi E, Modorati G, Foster CS (eds): New Treatments in Noninfectious Uveitis.
Dev Ophthalmol. Basel, Karger, 2012, vol 51, pp 98–109

Rituximab for Noninfectious Uveitis

Elisabetta Miserocchi · Giulio Modorati

Ocular Immunology and Uveitis Service, Department of Ophthalmology and Visual Sciences,
San Raffaele Scientific Institute, University Vita-Salute, Milan, Italy

Abstract

Rituximab (RTX) is a monoclonal antibody directed against the CD20 antigen expressed on B cells. This drug has been successfully employed in the treatment of non-Hodgkin's lymphoma and different systemic autoimmune diseases such as rheumatoid arthritis, systemic lupus erythematosus, granulomatosis with polyangiitis (Wegener's) and anti-neutrophil cytoplasmic antibody-associated vasculitis. At present, RTX may be used in patients with rheumatoid arthritis who qualify for treatment with tumor necrosis factor blockers and have had an inadequate response or intolerance to one or more of these agents. In ophthalmology, there is a growing amount of literature which suggests that RTX may be useful for inflammatory ocular diseases. Only few cases have been reported on treatment of ocular inflammatory disease mostly refractory scleritis, peripheral ulcerative keratitis, uveitis in adulthood and in children with juvenile idiopathic arthritis. RTX has also been employed in ocular surface diseases such as ocular cicatricial pemphigoid and conjunctival lymphoma. The tolerability and safety of RTX is good with the most common adverse events encountered being infusion reactions. RTX may be effective in the treatment of ocular inflammatory diseases, in particular the most aggressive, recalcitrant and sight-threatening forms of inflammation and uveitis. Although further studies are needed to assess the efficacy of RTX and the exact dosing regimen, RTX may be considered as a treatment alternative in patients with the most aggressive forms of inflammatory ocular diseases who fail to respond to conventional and other biologic agents.

Most forms of noninfectious uveitis have a chronic course, are recalcitrant to several treatments and are still associated with a high rate of visual loss.

The use of a wide range of drugs that control intraocular inflammation delays progression of visual impairment and improves the quality of life, but never brings about a complete cure. This failure has aroused an interest in new forms of experimental immunotherapy. Treatments employing monoclonal antibodies have made the most significant progress because they are based on consolidated experimental evidence since they have been used for more than 25 years. Moreover, advances in molecular biology have led to the identification of new immunotherapy target molecules, and biotechnology has produced modified (chimeric or humanized) monoclonal antibodies with a higher therapeutic index than the murine models. Rituximab (RTX), a monoclonal antibody to the anti-B cell-associated antigen CD20, is another valuable chimeric monoclonal antibody [1–3].

Approved by the FDA for the treatment of lymphomas, it has also attracted the interest of clinical immunologists because of the promising results it has achieved in the treatment of several autoimmune diseases [4].

RTX has been licensed for non-Hodgkin's lymphoma since 1997, and has been recently approved in United States and Europe for the treatment of patients with rheumatoid arthritis (RA) who have had inadequate response to tumor necrosis factor-α (TNF-α) blockers [4].

Little is known about the efficacy and tolerability of RTX treatment in patients with autoimmune ocular inflammatory diseases and in particular noninfectious uveitis.

Rituximab: General Considerations

Anti-CD20 RTX is a chimeric (murine and human) monoclonal antibody directed against the CD20 molecule, a tetraspan membrane protein found only on the surface of mature B cells [1–3, 5].

The CD20 molecule displays a dynamic appearance first evolving in the immature B cell stage and later disappearing when B cells differentiate into plasma cells. By targeting CD20, the killing of B cell precursor stem cells is avoided. Long-lived plasma cells residing in the bone marrow are also spared as most of them do not any longer carry the CD20 antigen. This means that immunoglobulin formation against isoantigens and antibodies against previously fought infectious agents are continuously formed. The mechanism with which RTX causes B cell death is not fully understood. It is, however, likely to be a combination of antibody-dependent cell-mediated cytotoxicity, complement-mediated lysis, growth inhibition and apoptosis. In vivo experiments using a mouse model of immunotherapy suggest that the most important mechanism of action is via antibody-dependent cell-mediated cytotoxicity [2]. The mechanisms do, however, work in a complex manner. For example, lymphoma cells of different maturation stages respond differently to RTX-induced apoptosis and inhibition of proliferation [1–3].

The rationale for a treatment aimed at B cell depletion is manifold: if autoantibody production is of pathogenetic significance, targeting the CD20 B cells prevents them from developing into autoantibody-producing plasma cells. However, long-lived plasma cells continue to secrete autoantibodies, and memory cells are probably not affected. Some patients develop reduction in their immunoglobulin levels, while some others do not. The reason for this discrepancy is not known. Another point could be that B cells are professional antigen-presenting cells, and the removal of B cells therefore prevents T cell activation [1–3, 5].

RTX was first approved by the FDA in 1997 for treatment of patients with relapsed or refractory lymphoma [4]. Since that time, its therapeutic range has gradually expanded to also include nonmalignant B cell-dependent diseases. Of these, rheumatoid arthritis (RA) is the autoimmune disease in which RTX has been most extensively studied [6–17].

The CD20 Antigen

CD20 antigen is a 33- to 35-kDa phosphoprotein expressed on B lymphocytes from the early pre-B to the late B stage, though its expression ceases when they differentiate into plasma cells.

The CD20's natural ligand has not been defined. Studies using specific monoclonal antibodies, however, have shown that this antigen is involved in B cell activation and proliferation by triggering tyrosine kinase intracellular signals and regulating intracellular calcium. CD20 engagement by the corresponding monoclonal antibody, in fact, blocks these functions and induces apoptosis, antibody-dependent cell-mediated cytotoxicity and complement-dependent cytotoxicity [2, 18].

These data, as well as the demonstration of CD20 on autoreactive B cells and recent indications that B cells have a broader pathogenetic role in the maintenance of autoreactive T cell activation, have led to the use of RTX for the treatment of autoimmune diseases [1, 2, 19, 20].

Rituximab in Systemic Autoimmune Diseases

Several clinical studies have demonstrated the substantial impact of RTX for treatment of various systemic autoimmune diseases [6–17]. Evidence of therapeutic effect is also mounting for numerous autoimmune conditions such as rheumatoid arthritis, systemic lupus erythematosus, granulomatosis with polyangiitis (Wegener's) and anti-neutrophil cytoplasmic antibody (ANCA)-associated vasculitis, idiopathic thrombocytopenic purpura, multiple sclerosis and Sjögren's syndrome [6–17]. A sustained B cell depletion of naïve and autoimmune cells is achieved, with peripheral blood CD20 cells being low or undetectable for up to 6 months, returning to pretreatment levels within 12 months. Earlier repopulation of B cells is observed after RTX monotherapy rather than after combination therapy with immunosuppressive agents, such as methotrexate [2].

Rituximab in Inflammatory Eye Diseases

Only a few publications have reported the effect of RTX on the course of severe immune-mediated inflammatory eye disease. Experience in the treatment of uveitis with RTX is still scarce with few case reports on its efficacy.

RTX has been successfully used in several forms of inflammatory diseases such as keratoconjunctivitis [16, 21], scleritis [22–26], peripheral ulcerative keratitis [27, 28], uveitis [29], juvenile idiopathic arthritis (JIA)-associated uveitis [30–32], retinal vasculitis [33–36].

Uveitis

RTX may be helpful in selected patients with chronic uveitis refractory to corticosteroid and conventional immunosuppressants. Tappeiner et al. [29] reported improvement of endogenous uveitis with cystoid macular edema in an adult patient treated with RTX; the treatment also had a steroid-sparing effect. However, in this reported case, the B cell depletion in the peripheral blood and the positive effect on uveitis was transient since there was a recurrence of inflammation after 6 and 9 months from RTX treatment.

Uveitis in Behçet's Disease

Ocular inflammation in Behçet's disease is believed to represent a CD4+ T cell and macrophage-mediated pathology, in which cell adhesion molecules, cytokines, oxygen free radicals and prostaglandins play an important role.

However, recently, conditions that are considered as predominantly T cell-mediated autoimmune diseases such as rheumatoid arthritis and granulomatosis with polyangiitis (Wegener's), have been treated successfully with RTX.

In addition to changes in number and activities of T cells, increased levels of activated and memory B cell subsets suggest a modified B cell function in Behçet's disease and certainly, B cell has a major role in T cell activity in addition to its role in antibody secretion [33].

Knowing that activated B lymphocytes are a source for IL-6, the use of RTX seems logical in patients with Behçet's uveitis since the level of IL-6 in the serum and in the aqueous humor of these patients is higher compared to normal controls [37].

Sadreddini et al. [35] were the first to report a case of retinal vasculitis in Behçet's disease treated with RTX; the patient had a complete remission of ocular inflammatory manifestations, and there were no relapses of vasculitis after the steroid-tapering period.

In another study by Davatchi et al. [34] comparing the efficacy of RTX versus other cytotoxic agents in 20 patients with retinal vasculitis in Behçet disease, the authors showed favorable results in the control of uveitis. In the present study, RTX was effective in the treatment of intractable ocular lesions of Behçet's disease, resistant to long-term cytotoxics and prednisolone. Results from the study of Davatchi et al. [34] are very interesting because they were obtained from patients with retinal vasculitis and macular edema who were nonresponders to cytotoxic drugs.

Uveitis in Children with Juvenile Idiopathic Arthritis

JIA is the most common systemic disorder associated with uveitis in childhood, accounting for approximately 75% of all pediatric anterior uveitis cases. Long-term ocular complications of uveitis such as cataract, band keratopathy, posterior synechia, glaucoma and maculopathy can lead to severe visual impairment in about 38% of patients [38]. Visual outcome in long-term follow-up of patients suffering from JIA-associated uveitis have been described as poor, with one third of patients developing substantial visual impairment and 10% becoming blind [39]. Aggressive immunomodulatory therapy is often introduced to improve the visual prognosis and reduce corticosteroid-induced adverse events [40]. With the advent of biologic agents, TNF-α antagonists have been successfully used and have changed and markedly improved the treatment options for JIA [41, 42]. However, a subset of patients fails to respond to TNF-α blockers or is unable to tolerate these therapies and may benefit from switching to another agent of this class or to a different biologic drug.

In a previous report on 10 patients with severe recalcitrant JIA-associated uveitis, we observed that RTX was capable of inducing inactivity in 7 patients [30]. Importantly, sparing of topical and systemic corticosteroids and associated immunosuppression was achieved after RTX infusions. Although the patients in this series had ongoing disease at an earlier stage, the good response after RTX suggests an important role of B cells in the pathogenesis of JIA uveitis. After one RTX cycle, sustained B cell depletion of naïve and autoimmune cells was achieved: peripheral blood CD20 cells were low or could not be detected for up to 6 months, returning to pretreatment levels within 12 months [30].

In 4 of these treated patients, the effect of RTX on uveitis was transient, with uveitis relapses occurring after 6–9 months after the first infusion. These relapses occurred in conjunction with B cell restoration, as CD19 cells were below detection level initially after RTX infusions and subsequently increased.

The lack of RTX efficacy in previous clinical trials on autoimmune disease has been attributed to the survival of long-lived autoreactive plasma cells, which do not harbor CD20 antigen.

The poor response to RTX in some of uveitis patients in this series may be related to the important role of plasma cells as the predominant producers of the antibodies.

No significant side effects from RTX were noted during the observation period in this small case series. However, the follow-up was relatively short.

Table 1. Previous and current treatment: previous and current immunosuppressants employed, previous anti-TNF employed, previous local and systemic corticosteroids employed

Patient no.	Immunosuppressants employed before RTX	Anti-TNF drugs employed before RTX	Immunosuppressants employed at last visit	Systemic steroid before RTX and at last visit (predniso-lone) mg/day	Topical steroids before RTX and at last visit daily frequency
1	MTX, CSA	Etan, Infl, Adal	none	7.5–0	3–1
2	MTX, CSA	Etan, Infl, Adal	none	25–12.5	4–1
3	MTX, CSA	Etan, Infl, Adal	none	0–0	4–2
4	MTX, CSA, AZA	Infl, Adal	CSA	25–12.5	3–1
5	MTX, CSA, CHLOR	Etan, Infl, Adal	MTX	20–12.5	6–0
6	MTX, CSA	Etan, Infl	none	15–0	2–0
7	MTX	Etan, Infl, Adal	MTX, CSA	0–0	2–1
8	MTX, CSA, CHLOR	Etan, Infl, Adal	none	20–2.5	2–1

MTX = Methotrexate; CSA = cyclosporine; CHLOR = chlorambucil; Etan = etanercept; Infl = infliximab; Adal = adalimumab.

We recently published our personal experience in treating patients with JIA-associated uveitis with RTX [31, 32].

We performed a retrospective analysis on 8 patients (2 males and 6 females; 14 affected eyes) with JIA-associated uveitis who received RTX therapy from July 2008 to November 2010.

RTX was given at the dose of 1,000 mg per infusion on days 1 and 15 and a recall 3rd infusion was scheduled at 12th and 21 months according to the rheumatologic protocol applied in the treatment of rheumatoid arthritis.

We achieved complete control of the uveitis with persistent clinical remission in 7 out of 8 patients at the end of follow-up. The decrease in uveitis activity was evident around the 4–5th month after the first infusion. Local and systemic corticosteroid-sparing effect of RTX was also noticeable in our patients; at the end of follow-up, 4 out of 6 patients taking systemic prednisolone were still on tapering daily low doses, but the dosage was significantly reduced compared to that needed at the beginning of RTX, and 2 patients discontinued systemic steroid therapy. Five out of 8 patients were also able to discontinue the concomitant systemic immunosuppressants.

None of the patients had a visual worsening during the follow-up and no serious adverse events were encountered in our treated patients (tables 1 and 2).

Uveitis Associated with Intraocular Lymphoma

Primary intraocular lymphoma is a hematopoietic tumor that arises within the retina, vitreous, subretinal pigment epithelial space or optic nerve head. Intraocular

Table 2. Clinical response to RTX, follow-up and visual acuity data, dose and number of RTX infusions

Patient no.	Activity of uveitis at last visit	Recurrence of uveitis, months from first infusion	Follow-up time on RTX months	Visual acuity before RTX	Visual acuity at last visit	RTX infusions (1,000-mg dose at each infusion)
1	no	10	25	20/40; NLP	20/40; NLP	3
2	no	no	23	20/40; 20/200	20/40; 20/40	3
3	yes	8, 21	21	20/20; 20/20	20/20; 20/20	4
4	no	no	14	20/20; 20/25	20/20; 20/25	3
5	no	no	11	20/60; 20/40	20/60; 20/40	2
6	no	no	10	20/20; NLP	20/20; NLP	2
7	no	no	8	20/20; 20/20	20/20; 20/20	3
8	no	no	7	NLP; 20/60	NLP; 20/60	2

NLP = No light perception.

lymphoma may manifest with different forms of uveitis called 'masquerade syndrome'. The malignancy is considered a subset of primary central nervous system lymphoma, which is a variant of extranodal non-Hodgkin lymphoma. Malignant lymphocytes present in intraocular lymphoma express certain B cell markers including CD20 [43]. Therefore, intraocular use of RTX has been explored in animal models for treatment of this condition. No ocular toxicity was found in rabbits and in humans treated with 1 mg of RTX injected in the vitreous cavity. Further studies are necessary to confirm the lack of toxicity at this dose and whether this local therapy is effective in eyes with intraocular lymphoma [43, 44].

Treatment of Other Ocular Inflammatory Diseases

Inflammation of the Sclera

Successful effectiveness with RTX has been reported in 3 patients with scleritis and peripheral ulcerative keratitis associated with granulomatosis with polyangiitis (Wegener's) [22, 24, 26]. Another case of peripheral ulcerative keratitis associated with granulomatosis with polyangiitis (Wegener's) that completely resolved with two RTX infusions given according to the rheumatologic protocol at the dose of 1,000 mg/infusion 2 weeks apart was described by Freidlin et al. [28]. Clinical improvement in 10 patients with refractory granulomatous ocular Wegener's mainly scleritis and orbital granulomas was reported by Taylor et al. [25]. Conversely, in another study the authors showed limited response of scleritis and orbital inflammation to RTX probably due to the presence of fibrotic nature of granulomas, especially when occurring in the retro-orbital region [45]. Ahmadi-Simab et al. [23] reported a case of refractory anterior scleritis associated with Sjögren's syndrome that completely resolved after four infusions of RTX given according to the oncologic protocol at the dose of 375 mg/m^2 at 4-week intervals.

Ocular Anti-Neutrophil Cytoplasmic Antibody-Associated Vasculitis

Taylor et al. [25] reported positive findings in 10 patients with ocular and orbital granulomatosis with polyangiitis (Wegener's) treated with RTX. All patients, had limited or incomplete responses to conventional treatment and had experienced numerous relapses and remissions associated with multiple side effects before treatment with RTX was initiated. In the present study, RTX induced remission of the disease in all 10 patients, and the effect was sustained for a median of 6.5 months, and for at least 12 months in 4 patients, without the need for additional treatment with corticosteroids or immunosuppressive medication. In this study, B cell depletion was associated with a trend toward decreased ANCA levels and clinical improvement in both vasculitic and granulomatous manifestations of the disease [25].

Persistence of ANCA production after RTX treatment in patients with ocular manifestations of granulomatosis with polyangiitis (Wegener's) might indicate either incomplete B cell depletion or the persistence of long-living plasma cells that are not affected by RTX because of their lack of CD20 expression. There is evidence that such plasma cells are an important source of autoantibodies in autoimmune disease. Indeed, the existence of ANCAs despite cytotoxic treatment in patients with Wegener's and the persistence of normal immunoglobulin levels after treatment with RTX imply the existence of long-lived plasma cells [46].

Dry Eye and Sjögren's Syndrome

Preliminary experiences of RTX therapy in Sjögren syndrome patients suggest that patients with more residual exocrine gland function might better benefit from RTX treatment. Sicca syndrome responded much better in the patient's perspective than in clinical objective evaluation, with about half of the patients reporting an improvement in oral and ocular dryness, while objective tests (Schirmer test) remained unchanged or worsened in all the patients [15, 16]. Zapata et al. [21] reported improvement of dry eye condition and quality of life in 2 patients with severe keratoconjunctivitis refractory to conventional therapeutic approach, treated with RTX.

Improvement in submandibular flow rate, dry mouth score, IgM rheumatoid factors, fatigue, and health-related quality of life tests, was also observed in Sjögren's patients after treatment with RTX [15, 21].

Safety of Rituximab

According to the experience from the rheumatologic studies on treatment of rheumatoid arthritis and lymphoma, the safety profile of RTX seems to be good [10, 11, 47].

The majority of adverse effects with the use of RTX reported in the literature are mild and transient with the most frequent adverse events being infusion reactions (30–35% with the first infusion). Examples of infusion reactions include hypotension, hypertensive crisis, chills, and skin rash. In general, the incidence of infusion-related side effects was reduced in patients with rheumatoid arthritis compared to patients with lymphoma. Premedication using intravenous glucocorticoids (100 mg methylprednisolone) reduce both the incidence and the severity of these reactions [10, 11, 47].

Fleischmann showed that the proportion of patients who had an acute infusion reaction following their first RTX infusion decreased after subsequent courses [48].

The main concern with the use of RTX in the treatment of autoimmune diseases, especially when used with concomitant immunosuppressive therapy, is the high incidence of systemic infections, which can sometimes lead to fatal septicemia [8, 13, 47, 49, 50].

A systematic review of the literature by Salliot et al. [51] did not reveal a significant increase in the risk of serious infections during RTX therapy. In this meta-analysis, the incidence of serious infections was 2.3% in the RTX group and 1.5% in the placebo group. In these patients receiving RTX, serious infections were mainly respiratory tract bacterial infections and no opportunistic infections or tuberculosis occurred.

In the study by Fleischmann [48], the incidence rates of infections were stable across treatment courses and the most common serious infections reported were upper respiratory tract infections, urinary tract infections, but they were also commonly observed during the first 3 months and possibly associated with concomitant use of glucocorticoids during the infusion periods. Moreover, when interpreting data on the incidence of infections in RA treated with different drugs, we had to remember that rheumatoid arthritis itself may be associated with an increased risk of infections.

Serum sickness reactions occur more frequently in patients with autoimmune diseases. As RTX is a chimeric human/mouse antibody, human antichimeric antibodies (HACAs) may occur and have been reported in about 9.2% of patients with RA. These HACAs may be responsible for infusion reactions [13, 47].

In 2006, the FDA received reports of patients who developed fatal progressive multifocal leukoencephalopathy (PML), following RTX treatment for systemic lupus erythematosus [52]. Even though data are limited in RA, a careful surveillance for PML symptoms is recommended [52]. Finally, RTX has been frequently associated with hepatitis B virus reactivation in oncology while its hepatic safety in rheumatic diseases is still unknown [53].

Retreatment

Recent data support the possibility of long-term continuation of RTX therapy without significant increase in side effects and infection rates. A work of Popa et al. [54] on 36 patients with rheumatoid arthritis followed for 5 years has shown that repeated B lymphocyte depletion (up to 5 cycles, 89 overall cycles) over a 5-year period appears to be effective and well tolerated. The average duration of benefit per cycle was 15 months and the time to retreatment was 20 months. A recent open label extension study of 1,053 patients analyzed efficacy and safety of additional courses of RTX in rheumatoid arthritis. The study showed that the most appropriate retreatment period was 6–12 months [55].

Conclusions

In conclusion, RTX is a new therapeutic option that can expand the therapeutic armamentarium for treatment of the most severe and recalcitrant sight-threatening forms of intraocular inflammation as well as diseases not responsive to TNF-α-blocking agents.

RTX, a humanized monoclonal antibody targeted to CD20, has been used extensively for treating systemic lymphoma, rheumatoid arthritis and other autoimmune diseases.

Like other biologic agents, RTX does not cure the disease, and recurrences of inflammation, after variable periods of time of sustained clinical remission, are possible and may require retreatment.

Studies of RTX in larger numbers of patients are needed to better evaluate the efficacy, dosing regimen, and safety of this treatment in patients with inflammatory ocular diseases recalcitrant to previous conventional treatments.

References

1 Blank M, Shoenfeld Y: B cell targeted therapy in autoimmunity. J Autoimmun 2007;28:62–68.

2 Perosa F, Favoino E, Caragnano MA, et al: CD20: a target antigen for immunotherapy of autoimmune diseases. Autoimmun Rev 2005;4:526–531.

3 Reff ME, Carner K, Chambers KS, et al: Depletion of B cells in vivo by a chimeric mouse human monoclonal antibody to CD20. Blood 1994;83:435–445.

4 Smolen JS, Keystone EC, Emery P, et al: Consensus statement on the use of rituximab in patients with rheumatoid arthritis. Ann Rheum Dis 2007;66: 143–150.

5 Arkfeld DG: The potential utility of B cell-directed biologic therapy in autoimmune diseases. Rheumatol Int 2008;28:205–215.

6 Shaw T, Quan J, Totoritis MC: B cell therapy for rheumatoid arthritis: the rituximab (anti-CD20) experience. Ann Rheum Dis 2003;62:ii55–ii59.

7 De Vita S, Quartuccio L: Treatment of rheumatoid arthritis with rituximab: an update and possible indications. Autoimmun Rev 2006;5:443–448.

8 Kunkel L, Wong A, Maneatis T, et al: Optimizing the use of rituximab for treatment of B-cell non-Hodgkin's lymphoma: a benefit-risk update. Semin Oncol 2000;27:53–61.

9 Edwards JC, Szczepanski I, Szczepanski J, et al: Efficacy of B-cell targeted therapy with rituximab in patients with rheumatoid arthritis. N Engl J Med 2004;17:350.

10 Caporali R, Caprioli M, Bobbio-Pallavicini F, et al: Long term treatment of rheumatoid arthritis with rituximab. Autoimmun Rev 2009;8:591–594.

11 Emery P, Fleishmann R, Filipowicz A, et al: The efficacy and safety of rituximab in patients with active rheumatoid arthritis despite methotrexate treatment: results of a phase IIB randomized, double-blind, placebo-controlled, dose-ranging trial. Arthritis Rheum 2006;54:1390–1400.

12 Conti F, Perricone C, Ceccarelli F, Valesini G: Rituximab treatment of systemic lupus erythematosus in controlled trials and in clinical practice: two sides of the same coin. Autoimm Rev 2010;9: 716–720.

13 Stasi R, Stipa E, Del Poeta G, et al: Long-term observation of patients with anti-neutrophil cytoplasmic antibody-associated vasculitis treated with rituximab. Rheumatology 2006;45:1432–1436.

14 Eriksson P: Nine patients with anti-neutrophil cytoplasmic antibody-positive vasculitis successfully treated with rituximab. J Intern Med 2005;257: 540–548.

15 Tobon GJ, Pers JO, Youinou P, Saraux A: B cell-targeted therapies in Sjogren's syndrome. Autoimm Rev 2010;9:224–228.

16 Quartuccio L, Fabris M, Salvin S, et al: Controversies on rituximab therapy in Sjogren syndrome-associated lymphoproliferation. Int J Rheumatol 2009;10:1–8.

17 Garcia-Carrasco M, Jimenez-Hernandez M, Escarcega RO, et al: Use of rituximab in systemic lupus erythematosus: an update. Autoimmun Rev 2009;8:343–348.

18 Deans JP, Li H, Polyak MJ: CD20-mediated apoptosis: signalling through lipid rafts. Immunology 2002;107:176–182.

19 Kneitz C, Wilhelm M, Tony HP: Effective B cell depletion with rituximab in the treatment of autoimmune diseases. Immunobiology 2002;206:519–527.

20 Di Gaetano N, Cittera E, Nota R, et al: Complement activation determines the therapeutic activity of rituximab in vivo. J Immunol 2003;171:1581–1587.

21 Zapata LF, Agudelo LM, Paulo JD, Pineda R: Sjogren keratoconjuntivitis sicca treated with rituximab. Cornea 2007;26:886–887.

22 Onal S, Kazokoglu H, Koc A, Yavuz S: Rituximab for remission induction in a patient with relapsing necrotizing scleritis associated with limited Wegener's granulomatosis. Ocul Immunol Inflamm 2008;16:230–232.

23 Ahmadi-Simab K, Lamprecht P, Nolle B, et al: Successful treatment of refractory anterior scleritis in primary Sjogren's syndrome with rituximab. Ann Rheum Dis 2005;64:1087–1088.

24 Kurz PA, Suhler EB, Choi D, Rosenbaum JT: Rituximab for treatment of ocular inflammatory disease: a series of four cases. Br J Ophthalmol 2009; 93:546–548.

25 Taylor SRJ, Salama AD, Josjhi L, et al: Rituximab is effective in the treatment of refractory ophthalmic Wegener's granulomatosis. Arthritis Rheum 2009; 50:1540–1547.

26 Cheung CM, Murray PI, Savage CO: Successful treatment of Wegener's granulomatosis associated scleritis with rituximab. Br J Ophthalmol 2005;89: 1542.

27 Huerva V, Sanchez MC, Traveset A, et al: Rituximab for peripheral ulcerative keratitis with Wegener granulomatosis. Cornea 2010;29:708–710.

28 Freidlin J, Wong IG, Acharya N: Rituximab treatment for peripheral ulcerative keratitis associated with Wegener's granulomatosis. Br J Ophthalmol 2007;91:1414.

29 Tappeiner C, Heinz C, Specker C, Heilighenhaus A: Rituximab as a treatment option for refractory endogenous anterior uveitis. Ophthalmic Res 2007; 39:184–186.

30 Heiligenhaus A, Miserocchi E, Heinz C, et al: Treatment of severe uveitis associated with juvenile idiopathic arthritis with anti-CD20 monoclonal antibody (rituximab). Rheumatology 2011;50: 1390–1394.

31 Miserocchi E, Pontikaki I, Modorati G, et al: Rituximab for uveitis. Ophthalmology 2011;118: 223–224.

32 Miserocchi E, Pontikaki I, Modorati G, et al: Anti-CD20 monoclonal antibody (rituximab) treatment for inflammatory ocular diseases. Autoimm Rev 2011;11:35–39.

33 Davatchi F: New and innovative therapies for Behçet's disease. APLAR J Rheum 2004;7:141–145.

34 Davatchi F, Shams H, Rezaipoor M, et al: Rituximab in intractable ocular lesions of Behcet's disease; randomized single-blind control study (pilot study). Int J Rheum Dis 2010;13:246–252.

35 Sadreddini S, Noshad H, Molaeefard M, Noshad R: Treatment of retinal vasculitis in Behcet's disease with rituximab. Mod Rheumatol 2008;18:306–308.

36 Hickman RA, Denniston AK, Yee CS, et al: Bilateral retinal vasculitis in a patient with systemic lupus erythematosus and its remission with rituximab therapy. Lupus 2010;19:327–329.

37 Charteris DG, Barton K, McCartney AC, Lightman SL: CD4+ lymphocyte involvement in ocular Behcet's Diseases. Autoimmunity 1992;12:201–206.

38 Heiligenhaus A, Niewerth M, Ganser G, et al: Prevalence and complications of uveitis in juvenile idiopahic arthritis in a population-based nationwide study in Germany: suggested modification of the current screening guidelines. Rheumatology 2007;46:1015–1059.

39 Thorne JE, Woreta F, Kedhar SR, et al: Juvenile idiopathic arthritis-associated uveitis: incidence of ocular complications and visual acuity loss. Am J Ophthalmol 2007;143:840–846.

40 Miserocchi E, Baltatzis S, Ekong A, et al: Efficacy and safety of chlorambucil in intractable noninfectious uveitis: the Massachusetts Eye and Ear Infirmary experience. Ophthalmology 2002;109:137–142.

41 Saurenmann RK, Levin AV, Rose JB, et al: Tumour necrosis factor-α inhibitors in the treatment of childhood uveitis. Rheumatology 2006;45:982–989.

42 Rajaraman RT, Kimura Y, Li S, et al: Retrospective case review of pediatric patients with uveitis treated with infliximab. Ophthalmology 2006;113:308–314.

43 Kitzmann AS, Pulido JS, Mohney BG, et al: Intraocular use of rituximab. Eye 2007;21:1524–1527.

44 Ohguro N, Hashida N, Tano Y: Effect of intravitreous rituximab injections in patients with ocular lesions associated with central nervous system lymphoma. Arch Ophthalmol 2008;126:1002–1003.

45 Aries PM, Hellmich B, Voswinkel J, et al: Lack of efficacy of rituximab in Wegener's granulomatosis with refractory granulomatous manifestations. Ann Rheum Dis 2006;65:853–858.

46 Cambridge G, Leandro MJ, Edwards JC, et al: Serologic changes following B lymphocyte depletion therapy for rheumatoid arthritis. Arthritis Rheum 2003;48:2146–2154.

47 Kimby E: Tolerability and safety of rituximab (MabThera). Cancer Treat Rev 2005;31:456–473.

48 Fleischmann RM: Safety of biologic therapy in rheumatoid arthritis and other autoimmune diseases: focus on rituximab. Semin Arthritis Rheum 2009;38:265–280.

49 Tam C, Seymour JF, Brown M, et al: Early and late infectious consequences of adding rituximab to fludarabine and cyclophosphamide in patients with indolent lymphoid malignancies. Haematologica 2005;90:700–702.

50 Kong JSW, Teuber SS, Gershwin ME: Potential adverse events with biologic response modifiers. Autoimm Rev 2006;5:471–485.

51 Salliot C, Dougados M, Gossec L: Risk of serious infections during rituximab, abatacept and anakinra therapies for rheumatoid arthritis: meta-analyses of randomized placebo-controlled trials. Ann Rheum Dis 2009;68:25–32.

52 Calabrese LH, Molloy ES: Progressive multifocal leucoencephalopathy in the rheumatic diseases: assessing the risks of biological immunosuppressive therapies. Ann Rheum Dis 2008;67(suppl 3): iii64–iii65.

53 Sera T, Hiasa Y, Michitaka K, et al: Anti-HBs-positive liver failure due to hepatitis B virus reactivation induced by rituximab. Intern Med 2006;45: 721–724.

54 Popa C, Leandro MJ, Cambridge G, et al: Repeated B lymphocyte depletion with rituximab in rheumatoid arthritis over 7 years. Rheumatology 2007;46: 626–630.

55 Keystone E, Fleischmann R, Emery P, et al: Safety and efficacy of additional courses of rituximab in patients with active rheumatoid arthritis: an open-label extension analysis. Arthritis Rheum 2007;56: 3896–3908.

Elisabetta Miserocchi
Ocular Immunology and Uveitis Service
Department of Ophthalmology and Visual Sciences
Scientific Institute San Raffaele
University Vita-Salute
Via Olgettina 60, IT–20132 Milan (Italy)
Tel. +39 02 26433512, E-Mail miserocchi.elisabetta@hsr.it

Miserocchi E, Modorati G, Foster CS (eds): New Treatments in Noninfectious Uveitis.
Dev Ophthalmol. Basel, Karger, 2012, vol 51, pp 110–121

Intravitreal Injection Therapy in the Treatment of Noninfectious Uveitis

Giulio Modorati · Elisabetta Miserocchi

Ocular Immunology and Uveitis Service, Department of Ophthalmology and Visual Sciences, San Raffaele Scientific Institute, University Vita-Salute, Milan, Italy

Abstract

Uveitis is responsible for 5–20% of legal blindness in the United States and in Europe. In noninfectious uveitis, the most frequent uveitic complication that endangers sight is cystoid macular edema. Clinical characteristics, inflammation grading and visual acuity determine the choice of the correct therapy for each patient. We can utilize drugs either alone or in combination using different dosages and routes of administration. Intravitreal injection directly into the vitreous cavity leads to rapid therapeutic drug concentration in the retinal tissue and reduces systemic side effects. Intravitreally injected triamcinolone acetonide is the most powerful drug for the treatment of cystoid macular edema related to intraocular inflammation, but it also causes the most frequent and serious side effects. Due to the numerous side effects associated with the use of corticosteroids, there is a need to identify other anti-inflammatory agents with a better safety profile. Recent studies have demonstrated that intravitreal immunosuppressant injections of methotrexate or anti-VEGF agents may lead to fewer intraocular side effects, but also have a lower therapeutic activity for the reduction of macular edema. At present, intraocular anti-TNF-α drugs do not show promising results. As regards nonsteroidal anti-inflammatory drugs, further data are necessary to fully understand their efficacy and potential side effects.

Uveitis is associated with a great variety of inflammatory or infectious ocular diseases. This condition is responsible for 5–20% of legal blindness in the United States and in Europe. In noninfectious uveitis, the main causes of visual acuity reduction are macular edema, optic nerve inflammation and vitritis [1].

Clinical characteristics, inflammation grading and visual acuity, together with the clinician's clinical experience, determine the choice of the correct therapy for each patient. By choosing the best possible treatment, we aim to maximize the beneficial effects and minimize the possible side effects of the drugs. We can utilize drugs either alone or in combination, using different dosages and routes of administration. The choice is conditioned by the clinical characteristics of the disease, laterality, age, sex and the presence of comorbidities [1].

The structure of the eye is an important limiting factor. Indeed, the goal of drug delivery is to obtain and maintain drug concentration in intraocular tissues in order to have a therapeutic, but not a deleterious, effect. Due to the ocular barrier to drug penetration, it is important to carefully consider the effects of intrinsic target drugs, their distribution into the tissue and their elimination [2].

The Structure of the Eye

The choroid has a rich network of large- and small-diameter vessels. The endothelial cells of these vessels have large fenestrations that allow rapid molecular diffusion, thus permitting the treatment of choroidal diseases with systemic therapy.

The retina is separated from the blood by the blood-ocular barrier. More specifically, in the posterior segment we find the blood-retina barrier (BRB) and in the anterior segment the blood-aqueous barrier. Two parts of the BRB regulate drug diffusion from the bloodstream to the neural retina.

The outer part of the BRB is the retinal pigment epithelium (RPE) that separates the choroidal network from the neural retina. The RPE shows tight junctions that are a barrier for small molecules passing from choroidal tissue to the neural retina.

The inner part of the BRB consists of endothelial cells of the retinal vessels that are separated from the surrounding retinal tissue. Its capillaries are characterized by the thick basement membrane layer and surrounded by tight junction-linked endothelial cells. With this anatomic structure, the inner part of the BRB prevents unrestricted molecular diffusion between the vitreous-retinal compound and the bloodstream. This, however, represents a problem for the therapeutic approach to intraocular diseases, and has led scientists to bypass the BRB by means of innovative drug delivery methods [2–4].

Drug Delivery to the Posterior Segment

To obtain drug therapeutic concentration in the posterior segment of the eye, we can use various methods of administration that give very different results. Using the topical route, the posterior segment does not receive therapeutic drug concentration due to the blood-aqueous barrier, low corneal permeability and rapid drop drainage through the nasolacrimal ducts.

While systemic drug administration allows therapeutic concentration to easily reach the choroid, the BRB greatly reduces the vitreous-retinal concentration of the pharmacological agent. To improve retinal concentration, we have to use high dosages that may lead to potentially severe systemic side effects.

Periocular or subTenon injection is less invasive than intravitreal injection, but it is also less effective. Physical barriers such as the sclera, conjunctival lymphatic vessels, choroid, and the RPE (outer BRB) may reduce drug absorption into the eye and the intraocular concentration of the drug does not result constant.

Intravitreal injection of the drug therefore appears to be the ideal route to reach therapeutic concentration in the posterior segment without the risk of systemic side effects. The direct injection of drugs bypasses the blood ocular barrier and allows rapid pharmacological action into the retinal tissue. This condition might determine various pharmacological problems related to direct drug toxicity of the retinal tissue [2–7].

Intravitreal Injection

Intravitreal injection concentrates drugs into the vitreous cavity leading to rapid therapeutic drug concentration in the retinal tissue. The drug is eliminated in two ways: through the anterior chamber and the retinal tissue. The rate of elimination and tissue diffusion depends on the molecular drug dimension and vitreous consistency. Larger molecules can remain in the vitreous for several weeks, while a solution of molecules smaller than 500 Da generally has a retention half-life of 3 days. The viscoelastic gel structure of the vitreous may be seriously damaged in the elderly or following vitrectomy surgery. These conditions can influence the flow and, consequently, the concentration of the drug in the retinal tissue [2–7].

Intravitreal Injection Technique

After topical anesthesia (lidocaine) and eyelash cleaning with povidone-iodine, the lid speculum is applied. Topical antibiotics are normally used before and after intravitreal injection, but the risk of septic endophthalmitis is similar whether they are used or not. The rate of endophthalmitis after i.v. injection is low (0.02%), confirming the safety of this technique [8].

A povidone-iodine solution (5%) is applied to the eye, and the injection is carried out in the inferotemporal quadrant to reduce the risk of retinal detachment and visual axis interference.

The pharmacological agent is prepared in a 1-ml tuberculin syringe with a 30/32-gauge needle. The injection is performed through the pars plana into the middle vitreous. The injection must be carried out slowly and without interruption. The safest drug volume to inject is generally 100 µl.

After the injection, the removal of the needle must be slow, and a cotton-tipped applicator must push on the same site of the injection to reduce reflux [8, 9].

Some authors have shown that use of tunneled technique may significantly reduce reflux, and that 29/30-gauge needles guarantee less pain during injection [9].

Immunomodulators

Immunosuppressant drugs are routinely used in place of systemic steroids in autoimmune disease and in noninfectious uveitis [1]. Intravitreal immunosuppressant drug injection helps in reducing systemic side effects, ocular hypertension and cataract formation secondary to corticosteroids.

Intraocular Methotrexate

Methotrexate (MTX) is a competitive inhibitor of dihydrofolate, and systemic MTX is chronically used to treat noninfectious uveitis, sparing systemic steroid assumption [1].

In recent years, intravitreal injection of MTX has been widely used to treat intraocular lymphoma [10]. The dose used is 400 µg in 0.1 ml, which is well tolerated by retinal tissue and remains in therapeutic concentration for 48–72 h [10].

Deng et al. [11] showed that intravitreal MTX injection in rabbit eyes was less likely to provoke bacterial endophthalmitis or ocular hypertension than intravitreal steroid injection.

Recently, various authors have reported small series of uveitis patients treated with intravitreal MTX [12–14]. Hardwig et al. [12] showed that a dose of 400 µg appears to be well tolerated and had positive effects on the preservation of visual acuity.

Taylor et al. [13] in a pilot study of 15 patients with unilateral noninfectious uveitis reactivation or macular edema showed that intravitreal MTX (400 µg in 0.1 ml) can reduce macular edema and improve visual acuity like after steroid treatment. They also obtained a reduction in systemic therapy in some patients and the relapse of inflammation, which occurred after a median of 4 months, was successfully treated with a further MTX injection. Ocular side effects were rare and acceptable (transient corneal epitheliopathy). None of these 15 patients developed endophthalmitis or ocular hypertension. Drug activity on retinal inflammation was relatively fast and visual acuity improved in one week.

Bae and Lee [14] demonstrated that increased intraocular levels of IL-6, IL-8, vascular endothelial growth factor (VEGF) and monocyte chemotactic protein 1 may be responsible for refractory retinal vasculitis in Behçet disease. Intravitreal MTX injection was effective and well tolerated even in steroid responders with refractory retinal vasculitis due to Behçet disease. Intravitreal MTX injection was associated with a significant reduction in IL-6 and IL-8 levels.

In a pilot study, Palakurthi et al. [15] evaluated the toxicity of a biodegradable microneedle implant loaded with MTX as a sustained release device in normal rabbit eyes. They demonstrated that this sustained release implant containing MTX was histopathologically nontoxic and well tolerated.

Intravitreal MTX injections might represent a therapeutic solution in those patients with unilateral posterior uveitis that cannot tolerate systemic steroid or immunosuppressant therapy, or are corticosteroid responders. In the future, further studies might clarify the role of this drug in local treatment (injection or device) of uveitis or uveitic macular edema.

Tacrolimus (FK506)

Tacrolimus (FK 506; Fujisawa Pharmaceutical Co, Japan) is a macrolide immunosuppressant that is more effective than cyclosporine in the liver, kidney and pulmonary transplantation. It also shows fewer systemic side effects than cyclosporine. Tacrolimus is effective when administered systemically in patients with refractory uveitis, but its effectiveness is limited due to the high incidence of severe adverse effects including nephrotoxicity, hypertension, hyperesthesia, muscular weakness, insomnia, tremor, photophobia, gastrointestinal symptoms and central nervous system alterations [16–19].

Many authors have evaluated the dose-related safety and efficacy of tacrolimus intravitreal injections in treating animal experimental autoimmune uveitis (EAU) [16–18].

Zhang et al. [19] treated EAU in Lewis rats with intravitreal injection of liposomes encapsulating tacrolimus (FK506). The treatment significantly reduces intraocular inflammation, and the drug remains in ocular fluids for 14 days. This study confirms that intravitreal injection of tacrolimus is highly active in controlling EAU in rats, and that liposome allowed tacrolimus to release gradually for 2 weeks, thus reducing the number of intraocular injections necessary to treat uveitis.

Anti-VEGF Drugs

Chronic intraocular inflammation is associated with increased production of inflammatory mediators, including VEGF, which are thought to disrupt the inner BRB of retinal vessels, resulting in subsequent macular edema [20].

This assumption justifies the use of intraocular anti-VEGF drugs to reduce macular edema and vascular inflammation. Intravitreal Anti-VEGF drugs are currently used to treat age-related subretinal neovascularization, diabetic macular edema, post-retinal vein occlusion edema. Many authors are now using these drugs to treat uveitic macular edema with ambiguous results [21–31].

Ranibizumab

Ranibizumab (Lucentis, Biotech) intravitreal injection is widely used in the treatment of age related subretinal neovascularization [21] and has also been used recently in inflammatory choroidal neovascularization [22].

Acharya et al. [23], in a case series of 7 uveitic patients, treated refractory macular edema with monthly ranibizumab intravitreal injections for 3 months. The conclusions of this study showed visual acuity improvement and macular edema regression. The same authors [24] recently described an observed therapeutic effect of ranibizumab in the untreated contralateral eyes of patients with bilateral uveitis-related cystoid macular edema (CME). They advocate further study to evaluate ranibizumab systemic viability after intravitreal injection.

Bevacizumab

Bevacizumab (Avastin, Genentech) is a recombinant humanized anti-VEGF monoclonal antibody that is widely used to treat age-related macular degeneration subretinal neovascularization [25].

Julian et al. [26] used intravitreal bevacizumab to treat subretinal neovascularization related to inflammatory diseases with transient results. Arevalo et al. [27] demonstrated that at 24-month follow-up, intravitreal bevacizumab improved visual acuity, and reduced macular edema in OCT and fluorescein angiography images.

Cordero Coma et al. [28] treated 13 patients with intravitreal bevacizumab (2.5 mg/0.1 ml) for macular edema secondary to uveitis. Their results too showed that the treatment is well tolerated and is associated with short-term visual acuity improvement and macular thickness reduction.

Other authors have shown similar results concerning the improvement of uveitic macular edema using bevacizumab intravitreal injection [29]. Lasave et al. [30] and Soheilian et al. [31] compared intravitreal injection of bevacizumab and triamcinolone acetonide to treat refractory uveitic macular edema. These two studies, with different length follow-ups, showed opposing results regarding visual acuity improvement.

Tumor Necrosis Factor -α Blockers

Tumor necrosis factor-α (TNF-α) is implicated in the pathogenesis of many chronic inflammatory diseases. TNF-α antagonists represent a significant advance in the treatment of many inflammatory diseases. The systemic utilization of these drugs in place of steroid treatment in autoimmune diseases is well defined. To avoid the systemic side effects of these drugs, some authors proposed local utilization with intraocular injection.

Adalimumab

Adalimumab (Humira, Abbott) is an anti-TNF constructed from a fully human monoclonal antibody. It is successfully used in the treatment of rheumatoid arthritis, psoriatic arthritis, ankylosing spondylitis, Crohn's disease, chronic psoriasis and juvenile idiopathic arthritis.

In ophthalmology, the systemic use of this drug obtained successful results in treating uveitis related to various autoimmune diseases [32–34].

Androudi et al. [35] evaluated the efficacy of a monthly adalimumab intraocular injection for refractory uveitis-related macular edema in 8 patients. The results did not show an improvement in visual acuity or CME reduction after 6 months of follow-up.

Infliximab

Infliximab (Remicade, Centocor) is a chimeric monoclonal antibody to TNF-α. It is currently used to treat rheumatoid arthritis, psoriatic arthritis, ankylosing spondylitis, Crohn's disease and psoriasis.

Infliximab has shown therapeutic effects for various types of uveitis related to systemic autoimmune diseases, particularly Behçet disease [36].

Many pilot studies demonstrated the safety of intraocular infliximab in animal models [37]. Farvardin et al. [38] treated 10 eyes of 7 patients with chronic persistent noninfectious uveitis and macular edema with intravitreal infliximab injections. They injected 1.5 mg/0.15 ml, and after 4 weeks of follow-up the study showed visual acuity improvement and macular thickness reduction.

In another study, Giganti et al. [39] demonstrated that low-dose (0.5 mg/0.5 ml) intravitreal infliximab was not well tolerated. They hypothesized the immunogenetic and retinotoxic effect of intravitreal infliximab.

Corticosteroids

Topical, periocular and intravitreal steroids and systemic steroids represent the gold standard for every new anti-inflammatory drug in the treatment of uveitis. In posterior uveitis with asymmetric disease or controlled uveitis with persistent macular edema, intravitreal steroids represent an important therapeutic option for the clinician [40].

Corticosteroids are the treatment cornerstone for uveitis and secondary macular edema. Treatment with corticosteroid intravitreal injections can achieve the desired predictable intraocular therapeutic concentrations [41]. They stabilize the BRB, reducing proinflammatory mediator production [42].

Intravitreal triamcinolone acetonide (IVTA) was first used by Machemer to reduce cellular proliferation after retinal detachment surgery in 1979 [43]. Triamcinolone acetonide is a water-insoluble steroid that is used in many fields of medicine. In ophthalmology, it can be administered into the subTenon or retrobulbar space, or directly into the vitreous [44].

Many authors used IVTA in various ocular pathologies related to systemic autoimmune disease. The main outcome of these studies was the reduction in intraocular inflammation and cystoid macular edema that were present despite systemic therapy. The results showed the efficacy, albeit temporary, of this treatment [45, 46].

Kok et al. [47] treated 54 patients with refractory CME with IVTA (4 mg) despite systemic and local treatment. After a mean follow-up of 8 months, 83% of treated eyes responded positively to the therapy with an improvement in visual acuity and a reduction of CME. After a mean of 4 weeks, 43.1% of treated eyes developed transient intraocular pressure (IOP) elevation that was greater than 10 mm Hg.

Many other studies have focused on the positive role of IVTA in the treatment of refractory CME caused by various inflammatory conditions secondary to ocular autoimmune disease, postradiation CME, immune-recovery uveitis, pseudophakic eyes and idiopathic CME [48–53]. Complications related to IVTA are well known, the most frequent being elevated IOP. Infective endophthalmitis, sterile endophthalmitis and cataract formation are less frequent [54].

Gillies et al. [55] in a double-blinded, placebo-controlled, randomized clinical trial tested the safety of a single IVTA. They described elevated IOP after IVTA as being the most common side effect. The increase in IOP occurred in about 30% of patients that require topical anti-glaucoma therapy. Eight months after the intravitreal injections, 71% of patients were able to discontinue the topical anti-glaucoma drops. Other studies showed IOP elevation in 40–50% of treated patients with most of them returning to a normal IOP after 13–17 months [56, 57]. The patients with the highest risk of IOP elevation are those under 40 years old with preexisting uveitis, higher baseline IOP or glaucoma [58].

Nonsteroidal Anti-Inflammatory Agents

Due to the numerous side effects associated with the use of corticosteroids, there is a need to identify other anti-inflammatory agents with a better safety profile. Recent studies have demonstrated the usefulness of nonsteroidal anti-inflammatory drugs (NSAIDs) as an alternative. NSAIDs are potent cyclooxygenase inhibitors and anti-inflammatory agents, with potential antiproliferative and antiangiogenic effects [59]. Unlike corticosteroids, NSAIDs are not associated with cataract formation or elevated IOP. Since the topical administration of NSAIDs does not deliver appreciable drug quantities to the posterior segment, intravitreal administration remains a viable option for treating inflammation of the posterior segment [59].

The NSAID diclofenac inhibits both the cyclooxygenase and lipoxygenase pathways. Although diclofenac has been used topically in the treatment of inflammatory conditions, intravitreal delivery has recently been under observation. Since diclofenac sodium is a low-molecular-weight drug, when in solution, as is the case with its commercial ophthalmic formulations, it is predicted to disappear rapidly from the vitreous humor, having a short half-life of 2.87 h. To maintain safe levels of diclofenac for prolonged periods in the eye, slow-release drug delivery systems, such as nanoparticles, microparticles, or implants, might be useful. Alternatively, the use of a suspension or a less soluble form of the drug might be useful in prolonging intravitreal drug delivery [59, 60].

Kim et al. reported nontoxic intraocular doses of two commercially available NSAIDs: ketorolac and diclofenac. They showed that 3,000 μg of ketorolac and 300 μg of diclofenac were nontoxic in the rabbit retina of the studied animals [61]. In another animal study, Baranano et al. [60] confirmed that a single intravitreal injection of diclofenac effectively reduces intraocular inflammation caused by lipopolysaccharide and prostaglandin production in rabbit eyes with uveitis.

Prostaglandins are one of the presumed causes of CEM in uveitis and after cataract surgery, or in diabetic macular edema. Intraocular ketorolac and diclofenac significantly inhibit prostaglandin production in animal models of uveitis. Given the established efficacy of topical NSAIDs in treating postsurgical macular edema, intraocular NSAIDs might offer a more potent treatment for this vision-threatening condition [60]. In a pilot study of intravitreal injection of diclofenac for the treatment of macular edema of various etiologies, one eye was affected by macular edema secondary to intermediate uveitis; this patient showed improved visual acuity and reduced central macular thickness during a 2-month follow up period after intravitreal injection of 500 μg/0.1 ml of diclofenac [62].

Larger studies are needed to evaluate the role of intraocular NSAIDs, including diclofenac, in different entities, to help define the ideal regimen, duration of treatment, potential of combination treatment, and the safety of long-term treatment.

References

1 de Smet MD, Taylor SR, Bodaghi B, Miserocchi E, Murray PI, Pleyer U, Zierhut M, Barisani-Asenbauer T, Lehoang P, Lightman S: Understanding uveitis: the impact of research on visual outcomes. Prog Retin Eye Res 2011;30:452–470.

2 Thrimawithana TR, Young S, Bunt CR, Green C, Alany RG: Drug delivery to the posterior segment of the eye. Drug Discov Today 2011;16:270–277.

3 Duvvuri S, Majumdar S, Mitra AK: Drug delivery to the retina: challenges and opportunities. Expert Opin Biol Ther 2003;3:45–56.

4 Kuppermann BD, Loewenstein A: Drug delivery to the posterior segment of the eye. Dev Ophthalmol 2010;47:59–72.

5 Lobo AM, Sobrin L, Papaliodis GN: Drug delivery options for the treatment of ocular inflammation. Semin Ophthalmol 2010;25:283–288.

6 Maurice D: Review: practical issues in intravitreal drug delivery. J Ocul Pharmacol Ther 2001;17: 393–401.
7 Yasukawa T, Tabata Y, Kimura H, Ogura Y: Recent advances in intraocular drug delivery systems. Recent Pat Drug Deliv Formul 2011;5:1–10.
8 Sampat KM, Garg SJ: Complications of intravitreal injections. Curr Opin Ophthalmol 2010;21:178–183.
9 Rodrigues EB, Grumann A Jr, Penha FM, Shiroma H, Rossi E, Meyer CH, Stefano V, Maia M, Magalhaes O Jr, Farah ME: Effect of needle type and injection technique on pain level and vitreal reflux in intravitreal injection. J Ocul Pharmacol Ther 2011;27: 197–203.
10 Pe'er J, Hochberg FH, Foster CS: Clinical review: treatment of vitreoretinal lymphoma. Ocul Immunol Inflamm 2009;17:299–306.
11 Deng SX, Penland S, Gupta S, Fiscella R, Edward DP, Tessler HH, Goldstein DA: Methotrexate reduces the complications of endophthalmitis resulting from intravitreal injection compared with dexamethasone in a rabbit model. Invest Ophthalmol Vis Sci 2006;47:1516–1521.
12 Hardwig PW, Pulido JS, Erie JC, Baratz KH, Buettner H: Intraocular methotrexate in ocular diseases other than primary central nervous system lymphoma. Am J Ophthalmol 2006;142:883–885.
13 Taylor SR, Habot-Wilner Z, Pacheco P, Lightman SL: Intraocular methotrexate in the treatment of uveitis and uveitic cystoid macular edema. Ophthalmology 2009;116:797–801.
14 Bae Jh, Lee SC: Effect of intravitreal methotrexate and aqueous humor cytokine levels in refractory retinal vasculitis in Behçet disease. Retina 2011, Epub ahead of print.
15 Palakurthi NK, Correa ZM, Augsburger JJ, Banerjee RK: Toxicity of a biodegradable microneedle implant loaded with methotrexate as a sustained release device in normal rabbit eye: a pilot study. J Ocul Pharmacol Ther 2011;27:151–156.
16 Li S, Tang S, Li W, Li D Yan Ke Xue Bao: Experiment study of retinal ultrastructure after intravitreal FK506. Yan Ke Xue Bao 2004;20:34–38.
17 Ishikawa T, Hokama H, Katagiri Y, Goto H, Usui M: Effects of intravitreal injection of tacrolimus (FK506) in experimental uveitis. Eye Res 2005;30: 93–101.
18 Oh-i K, Keino H, Goto H, Yamakawa N, Murase K, Usui Y, Kezuka T, Sakai J, Takeuchi M, Usui M: Intravitreal injection of tacrolimus (FK506) suppresses ongoing experimental autoimmune uveoretinitis in rats. Br J Ophthalmol 2007;91:237–242.
19 Zhang R, He R, Qian J, Guo J, Xue K, Yuan YF: Treatment of experimental autoimmune uveoretinitis with intravitreal injection of tacrolimus (FK506) encapsulated in liposomes. Invest Ophthalmol Vis Sci 2010;51:3575–3582.
20 Fine HF, Baffi J, Reed GF, Csaky KG, Nussenblatt RB: Aqueous humor and plasma vascular endothelial growth factor in uveitis-associated cystoid macular edema. Am J Ophthalmol 2001;132:794–796.
21 Patel RD, Momi RS, Hariprasad SM: Review of ranibizumab trials for neovascular age-related macular degeneration. Semin Ophthalmol 2011;26: 372–379.
22 Rouvas A, Petrou P, Douvali M, Ntouraki A, Vergados I, Georgalas I, Markomichelakis JN: Intravitreal ranibizumab for the treatment of inflammatory choroidal neovascularization. Ocul Pharmacol Ther 2011;27:197–203.
23 Acharya NR, Hong KC, Lee SM: Ranibizumab for refractory uveitis-related macular edema. Am J Ophthalmol 2009;148:303–309.
24 Acharya NR, Sittivarakul W, Qian Y, Hong KC, Lee SM: Bilateral effect of unilateral ranibizumab in patients with uveitis related macular edema. Retina 2011;31:1871–1876.
25 El-Mollayess GM, Noureddine BN, Bashshur ZF: Bevacizumab and neovascular age related macular degeneration: pathogenesis and treatment. Semin Ophthalmol 2011;26:69–76.
26 Julián K, Terrada C, Fardeau C, Cassoux N, Français C, LeHoang P, Bodaghi B: Intravitreal bevacizumab as first local treatment for uveitis-related choroidal neovascularization: long-term results. Acta Ophthalmol 2011;89:179–184.
27 Arevalo JF, Adan A, Berrocal MH, Espinoza JV, Maia M, Wu L, Roca JA, Quiroz-Mercado H, Ruiz-Moreno JM, Serrano MA: Intravitreal bevacizumab for inflammatory choroidal neovascularization: results from the Pan-American Collaborative Retina Study Group at 24 months. Pan-American Collaborative Retina Study Group. Retina 2011;31: 353–363.
28 Cordero Coma M, Sobrin L, Onal S, Christen W, Foster CS: Intravitreal bevacizumab for treatment of uveitic macular edema. Ophthalmology 2007;114: 1574–1579.
29 Lott MN, Schiffman JC, Davis JL: Bevacizumab in inflammatory eye disease. Am J Ophthalmol 2009; 148:711–717.
30 Lasave AF, Zeballos DG, El-Haig WM, Díaz-Llopis M, Salom D, Arevalo JF: Short-term results of a single intravitreal bevacizumab (avastin) injection versus a single intravitreal triamcinolone acetonide (kenacort) injection for the management of refractory noninfectious uveitic cystoid macular edema. Ocul Immunol Inflamm 2009;17:423–430.

31 Soheilian M, Rabbanikhah Z, Ramezani A, Kiavash V, Yaseri M, Peyman GA: Intravitreal bevacizumab versus triamcinolone acetonide for refractory uveiti cystoid macular edema: a randomized pilot study. J Ocul Pharmacol Ther 2010;26:199–206.
32 Erckens RJ, Mostard RL, Wijnen PA, Schouten JS, Drent M: Adalimumab successful in sarcoidosis patients with refractory chronic non-infectious uveitis. Graefes Arch Clin Exp Ophthalmol 2011, Epub ahead of print.
33 Olivieri I, Leccese P, D'Angelo S, Padula A, Nigro A, Palazzi C, Coniglio G, Latanza L: Efficacy of adalimumab in patients with Behçet's disease unsuccessfully treated with infliximab. Clin Exp Rheumatol 2011;29(suppl 67):S54–S57.
34 Kotaniemi K, Säilä H, Kautiainen H: Long-term efficacy of adalimumab in the treatment of uveitis associated with juvenile idiopathic arthritis. Clin Ophthalmol 2011;5:1425–1429.
35 Androudi S, Tsironi E, Kalogeropoulos C, Theodoridou A, Brazitikos P: Intravitreal adalimumab for refractory uveitis-related macular edema. Ophthalmology 2010;117:1612–1616.
36 Handa T, Tsunekawa H, Yoneda M, Watanabe D, Mukai T, Yamamura M, Iwaki M, Zako M: Long-term remission of ocular and extraocular manifestations in Behçet's disease using infliximab. Clin Exp Rheumatol 2011;29(suppl 67):S58–S63.
37 Hosseini H, Safaei A, Khalili MR, Nowroozizadeh B, Eghtedari M, Farvardin M, Nowroozizadeh S, Tolide-Ie HR: Intravitreal infliximab in experimental endotoxin-induced uveitis. Eur J Ophthalmol 2009;19:818–823.
38 Farvardin M, Afarid M, Mehryar M, Hosseini H: Intravitreal infliximab for the treatment of sight-threatening chronic noninfectious uveitis. Retina 2010;30:1530–1535.
39 Giganti M, Beer PM, Lemanski N, Hartman C, Schartman J, Falk N: Adverse events after intravitreal infliximab (Remicade). Retina 2010;30:71–80.
40 Siddique SS, Shah R, Suelves AM, Foster CS: Road to remission: a comprehensive review of therapy in uveitis. Expert Opin Investig Drugs 2011;20:1497–1515.
41 de Smet MD, Okada AA: Cystoid macular edema in uveitis. Dev Ophthalmol 2010;47:136–147.
42 Edelman JL, Lutz D, Castro MR: Corticosteroids inhibit VEGF-induced vascular leakage in a rabbit model of blood-retinal and blood-aqueous barrier breakdown. Exp Eye Res 2005;80:249–258.
43 Machemer R, Sugita G, Tano Y: Treatment of intraocular proliferations with intravitreal steroids. Trans Am Ophthalmol Soc 1979;7:171–178.
44 Taylor SR, Isa H, Joshi L, Lightman S: New developments in corticosteroid therapy for uveitis. Ophthalmologica 2010;224(suppl 1):46–53.
45 Peyman GA, Lad EM, Moshfeghi DM: Intravitreal injection of therapeutic agents. Retina 2009;29:875–912.
46 Tao Y, Jonas JB: Intravitreal triamcinolone. Ophthalmologica 2011;225:1–20.
47 Kok H, Lau C, Maycock N, McCluskey P, Lightman S: Outcome of intravitreal triamcinolone in uveitis. Ophthalmology 2005;112:1916, e1–e7.
48 Antcliff RJ, Spalton DJ, Stanford MR, Graham EM, Ffytche TJ, Marshall J: Intravitreal triamcinolone for uveitic cystoid macular edema: an optical coherence tomography study. Ophthalmology 2001;108:765–772.
49 Martidis A, Duker JS, Puliafito CA: Intravitreal triamcinolone for refractory cystoid macular edema secondary to birdshot retinochoroidopathy. Arch Ophthalmol 2001;119:1380–1383.
50 Jonas JB, Kreissig I, Degenring RF: Intravitreal triamcinolone acetonide for pseudophakic cystoid macular edema. Am J Ophthalmol 2003;136:384–386.
51 Sutter FK, Gillies MC: Intravitreal triamcinolone for radiation-induced macular edema. Arch Ophthalmol 2003;121:1491–1493.
52 Sirimaharaj M, Robinson MR, Zhu M, Csaky KG, Donovan B, Sutter F, Gillies MC: Intravitreal injection of triamcinolone acetonide for immune recovery uveitis. Retina 2006;26:578–580.
53 Scott IU, Flynn HW Jr, Rosenfeld PJ: Intravitreal triamcinolone acetonide for idiopathic cystoid macular edema. Am J Ophthalmol 2003;136:737–739.
54 Sampat KM, Garg SJ: Complications of intravitreal injections. Curr Opin Ophthalmol 2010;21:178–183.
55 Gillies MC, Simpson JM, Billson FA, Luo W, Penfold P, Chua W, Mitchell P, Zhu M, Hunyor AB: Safety of an intravitreal injection of triamcinolone: results from a randomized clinical trial. Arch Ophthalmol 2004;122:336–340.
56 Jonas JB, Kreissig I, Degenring R: Intraocular pressure after intravitreal injection of triamcinolone acetonide. Br J Ophthalmol 2003;87:24–27.
57 Jonas JB, Kreissig I, Degenring R: Intravitreal triamcinolone acetonide for treatment of intraocular proliferative, exudative, and neovascular diseases. Prog Retin Eye Res 2005;24:587–611.
58 Sallam A, Taylor SR, Lightman S: Review and update of intraocular therapy in noninfectious uveitis. Curr Opin Ophthalmol 2011;22:517–522.

59 Durairaj C, Kim SJ, Edelhauser HF, Shah JC, et al: Influence of dosage from on the intravitreal pharmacokinetics of diclofenac. Invest Ophthalmol Vis Sci 2009;50:4887–4897.
60 Baranano DE, Kim SJ, Edelhauser HF, Durairaj C, et al: Efficacy and pharmacokinetics of intravitreal non-steroidal anti-inflammatory drugs for intraocular inflammation. Br J Ophthalmol 2009;93:1387–1390.
61 Kim SJ, Adams NA, Toma HS, Belair ML, et al: Safety of intravitreal ketorolac and diclofenac: an electroretinographic and histopathologic study. Retina 2008;28:595–605.
62 Soheilian M, Karimi S, Ramezani A, Peyman GA: Pilot study of intravitreal injection of diclofenac for treatment of macular edema of various etiologies. Retina 2010;30:509–515.

Giulio Modorati, MD
Ocular Immunology and Uveitis Service
Department of Ophthalmology and Visual Sciences
Scientific Institute San Raffaele
University Vita-Salute
Via Olgettina 60
IT–20132 Milan (Italy)
Tel. +39 02 26433565, E-Mail modorati.giulio@hsr.it

Miserocchi E, Modorati G, Foster CS (eds): New Treatments in Noninfectious Uveitis.
Dev Ophthalmol. Basel, Karger, 2012, vol 51, pp 122–133

Corticosteroid Intravitreal Implants

Marc D. de Smet

Retina and Inflammation, MIOS, Lausanne, Switzerland, and Department of Ophthalmology,
University of Amsterdam, Amsterdam, The Netherlands

Abstract

Intraocular implants developed for ocular inflammation which release glucocorticoids for a prolonged period within the vitreous cavity make use of either a bioerodible polymer (dexamethasone in polylactic acid-coglycolic acid matrix) or non-erodible implantable device (fluocinolone acetonide, FA, in a polyvinyl acetate/silicone laminate). Pharmacologically, both steroids are similar in their binding characteristics to glucocorticoid receptors (GR), their ability to transactivate the GR complex and their vitreous half-lives. They both possess neuroprotective properties for retina and retinal pigment epithelium which place them apart from triamcinolone acetonide. Triamcinolone acetonide's higher lipophilicity makes it possible to create an implant with prolonged release characteristics, but may be increasing the propensity for ocular side effects such as cataract and glaucoma. In clinical trials, both implants were shown to be effective at inhibiting intraocular inflammation in patients with intermediate or posterior uveitis. The Dexamethasone implant is inserted through a 22-gauge needle through the pars plana and can control inflammation for up to 6 months. The FA implant requires surgical insertion through the pars plana and can control inflammation for up to 3 years. The MUST trial has shown the FA implant when placed bilaterally to be slightly more effective than strict systemic therapy, though at the cost of additional ocular surgeries for cataract and glaucoma. Certain clinical situations particularly with asymmetric uveitis may in fact favor local vs. systemic therapy.

Ocular inflammation can be controlled by either local therapy or by way of systemically administered medication. While specific guidelines on the use of systemic steroids were published in 2000 suggesting that doses above 10 mg/day be used for 3 months or less, a recent survey among specialists treating uveitis in the United States showed that the majority did not abide by these guidelines [1, 2]. The frequency of adverse events due to immunosuppression in this study was high, 42 and 45% for posterior uveitis and panuveitis, respectively. Local treatment has the advantage of minimizing systemic side effects while allowing the administration of much higher concentrations of medication close to the desired site of action. While periocular steroids can provide therapeutic intraocular levels, there is often a delayed and variable response [3, 4]. Slow-release intraocular implants have definite advantages over more conventional approaches as the effect can be sustained for a prolonged period of time while minimizing both systemic uptake and side effects. It may also allow for a more judicious choice of steroid, one with an appropriate profile between potency, solubility, and side effects.

Pharmacology of Steroids

Glucocorticoids (GC) are at the apex of a regulatory network that blocks several inflammatory pathways including: eicosanoid synthesis (via annexin I); release and mediation by cytokines, chemotactic proteins and matrix metalloproteinases (via MAPK phosphatase 1 and IκB kinases); secretion of inflammatory proteins such as VEGF and cyclooxygenase 2 by reducing the stability of their mRNA [5]. Steroids mediate their effects via GC receptors (GR). Within the cytosol, GC bind to GR with high affinity, and mediate their action in three ways. Cytosolic GC-GR complex (GGR) acts through membrane-associated receptors through nongenomic activation. Within the nucleus, GGR forms homodimers which bind directly to specific DNA sequences forming GC-responsive complexes facilitating or repressing DNA transcription (direct genomic effect), or bond to other DNA protein complexes thereby modifying their signal (indirect genomic effect) such as NF-κB nuclear elements. Experimentally, direct genomic effects require fairly high concentrations of GC, while the indirect genomic effects can occur at somewhat lower concentrations [5, 6]. GR exists in several isoforms, some of which are more prone to act within the cytosol (hGR-α) or/and bind to specific nuclear motifs (hGR-α or hGR-β) [6, 7]. Their binding affinity for various GC varies. Their synthesis depends on the specific genetic make-up of the patient, his state of immune activation, and cell type.

Modifying the structure of a steroid modifies its biologic activity and its ability to bind to GR. In the past, the classification of GC was based on relative potency, determined in large part by a skin blanching test obtained by dissolving the steroids in alcohol and applying it to exposed skin [8, 9]. The potency of a given corticosteroid might be better assessed by taking into account its GR-binding affinity and gene transactivation. When comparing the three most commonly used intraocular steroids, dexamethasone (DEX), fluocinolone acetonide (FA), and triamcinolone acetonide (TA), GR-binding affinities are roughly equivalent (DEX 5.4 nM, FA 2.0 nM, TA 1.5 nM) [10]. Their potencies in transactivating GR are also equivalent when tested in a GeneBLAzer assay using HeLa cells. Plasma elimination half-lives for these three compounds vary; however, the vitreous elimination half-lives do not [7]. The solubilized fraction is rapidly cleared from the vitreous with an elimination half-life of 2–3 h. For an extended duration of action, this rapid clearance from the vitreous mandates that fresh compound be provided whether by dissolution of crystals or by controlled delivery from a reservoir.

Patient responses to GC vary significantly. These differences among patients and also between different cell types are believed to be linked to the unique hGR-α distribution in cells and their ability to bind to GC. There is evidence that different GC can generate a set of common and unique genes in relevant ocular tissues [10, 11]. Therefore, the therapeutic index of individual steroids will depend on the exact profile of the genes that are expressed or repressed. DEX and FA have been shown to exhibit neuroprotective effects in animal models of retinitis pigmentosa [12, 13]. By opposition, TA causes retinal toxicity by nonapoptotic, caspase-independent cell death [14, 15]. Differential response profiles for GC on different ocular tissue structures are still rare, but their availability may help guide the choice of GC for particular applications.

Design and Pharmacology of Steroid Implants

Implants come in basically two types – bioerodible polymers and inert shells which slowly release drug. With current available technologies and implantable steroids, the former are easier to insert but the duration of action is shorter. Both are effective at inhibiting ocular inflammation. Bioerodible polymers have been on the market for a short period of time, and clinical studies were carried out for relatively short intervals compared to the steroid implants. Therefore, it is difficult to compare long-term outcomes, and rates of ocular complications. However, DEX appears to cause less severe IOP increases, and possibly less cataract [16]. The peak in cataract incidence for cataract surgery following TA implants was between 12 and 24 months following surgery. Further studies will be required to elucidate this issue for DEX implants.

DEX was formulated in a solid biodegradable polymer composed of a polylactic acid-coglycolic acid (PLGA) matrix. The PLGA polymer matrix dissolves completely in vivo into its components, lactic acid and glycolic acid, which are in turn converted into carbon dioxide and water. As the polymer dissolves, DEX is released to its target tissues, the retina and vitreous over a 6-month period [17, 18]. The commercial preparation Osurdex (Allergan Inc, Irvine CA) contains 700 μg of DEX and was formulated to be administered via a 22-gauge injecting applicator through the pars plana similar to other intravitreal injections. The application is performed under sterile technique using a bi-planar injection. Using mass spectrometry and expression of the DEX-sensitive gene cytochrome P450 A38 (CYP3A8), the pharmacology and pharmacokinetics of Osurdex was determined [18]. Thirty-four male monkeys received bilateral 0.7 mg DEX implants; 3 animals served as controls. Samples of blood, vitreous, and retina were retrieved up to 270 days after initial implantation. DEX was detectable in the retina and vitreous for 6 months after administration. The peak concentration of DEX was reached in the retina and vitreous at day 60 (1,110 ± 284 ng/g and 213 ± 49 ng/ml, respectively). There was minimal systemic absorption with a peak concentration of 1.11 ng/ml in the serum at 2 months. Following the first

2 months, there was a steady decline in steroid concentration from month 2 to month 4, after which a second steady state was achieved and maintained until month 6 (day 180, retina DEX level: 0.0167 ± 0.0193 ng/g, vitreous level: 0.00131 ± 0.00194 ng/ml). The CYP3A8 expression increased more than 3-fold in eyes that had received the implant compared to control eyes, and this increased expression was sustained for 6 months. The pharmacokinetic profile of the implant was also compared between vitrectomized and nonvitrectomized eyes and found to be similar. Several drugs such as VEGF, triamcinolone, and amphotericin are cleared more rapidly in vitrectomized eyes [19–21]. A more rapid clearance of drug from the vitreous cavity can potentially affect the clinical effectiveness of these drugs as observed in macular edema and selected patients with AMD.

Fluocinolone has been incorporated in implantable nonbiodegradable sustained delivery devices. The Retisert (Bausch & Lomb) contains a 2-mg pellet of FA surrounded by a polyvinyl acetate/silicone laminate fixed onto a strut [22]. Through a central diffusion port, the GC leaches out in a linear fashion for up to 3 years (zero order kinetics) [23, 24]. It is implanted through a sclerotomy incision made at the level of the pars plana and is secured with a suture to the sclera. These implants were placed in 24 New Zeland black/satin rabbits and followed for up to one year. At various time points, levels of FA were measured in ocular tissue and blood. Ocular drug levels were stable over a year, and averaged 106 ± 18 ng/g for the vitreous and 336 ± 43 ng/g in the retina [23]. Comparable levels were also detected in the lens (296 ± 34 ng/g), the iris-ciliary body (178 ± 24 ng/g), and the retinal pigment epithelium (138 ± 26 ng/g). There was no evidence of systemic absorption. There are no data on the release rates in vitrectomized eyes; however, as with Osurdex, these are probably stable. An interesting experiment in rabbits looked at vitreous levels in gas-filled eyes following implantation of a sustained release implant containing a codrug consisting in FA and 5-fluorouracil in a 1:1 M ratio. Half of the animals had a 0.4 ml 100% C_3F_8 gas bubble injected in the mid-vitreous following implantation. The presence of the intraocular gas did not significantly affect the intravitreal drug levels during the 42 days of the study [25].

FA has also been formulated in the shape of a long sustained release tube that can be injected into the vitreous cavity through a 25-gauge needle. Iluvien (Alimera Science) is designed to release a 180-µg cylindrical pellet at a rate of either 0.2 or 0.5 µg per day at near-zero order kinetics for 2–3 years depending on the release rates [26, 27]. Both devices in a human DME trial showed sustained levels in the aqueous of between 1.5 and 2.4 ng/ml at one year, irrespective of the implant used [27].

In all delivery systems so far, placement has been aimed at the pars plana. Drug distribution from this location appears to be directed mainly at the posterior pole with a decreasing drug gradient existing between the site of implantation and the posterior retina [28, 29]. Little distribution of drug into the anterior segment was seen using Gd-DTPA intravitreal implants when imaged by MRI [28]. However, as indicated for the Retisert implant, FA levels comparable to the vitreous can be detected in the lens and ciliary body. Binding of GC to the lens and trabecular meshwork appears to be dependent on the lipophilicity of the GC (FA>TA>DEX) [30]. Certainly the rate of cataract formation and glaucoma seem to follow this trend [16, 30]. GR is present in both the lens and trabecular meshwork, and upon binding with GC leads to the activation of certain gene clusters [31, 32]. It is possible that differential rates of cataract formation or the incidence of steroid-induced glaucoma are related to the amount of GC taken up by these tissues. In an ex vivo model, at physiologic pH, all GC showed a preferential accumulation in bovine trabecular meshwork but partition coefficients for FA and TA were 1.85- and 1.56-fold higher than for DEX [30]. The lens partition coefficients were also higher for FA and TA (1.53- and 1.44-fold) as compared to DEX, but were overall lower than for the trabecular meshwork. There is a suggestion, which requires further evaluation, by which the partition coefficients increase as the lens ages.

Clinical Efficacy and Tolerability of Steroid Intravitreal Implants

Published phase III trials were carried out with the Ozurdex implant to treat retinal vein occlusion, diabetic macular edema and uveitis patients [33–35]. Patients with vision loss due to macular edema secondary to retinal vein occlusion were eligible for inclusion in a study randomizing in a 1:1:1 ratio to either sham procedure or treatment with DEX intravitreal implant at 0.35- and 0.7-mg dose. The study included 1,267 patients and demonstrated that the percentage of eyes achieving 15-letter improvement was significantly greater in both DEX-treated groups compared to sham [33]. The greatest response was seen at day 60 in the 0.7-mg implant group with 29% of patients achieving 15-letter improvement. Cataracts were not increased in any group. 16% of implanted eyes had an increase in IOP that was greater than 15 mm Hg. Whereas 30% of eyes were treated with IOP-lowering medication at day 90, the IOP returned to baseline by day 180 in all groups. Five eyes required a surgical intervention for IO control, and 3 of these were for neovascular glaucoma. At the end of 180 days, all patients with a drop in vision under 20/20 or OCT thickness >250 μm were eligible to receive a 0.7-mg DEX implant. The side effect profile was similar in the open-label extension except that over 12 months, cataract progression in those patients receiving 2 implants was observed in 90/302 (29.8%) of phakic eyes as compared to 5/88 (5.7%) of sham-treated eyes [36]. Only one patient required cataract surgery.

Lowder et al. [35] evaluated the efficacy of 0.35 and 0.7 mg DEX intravitreal implant compared to sham in 229 patients diagnosed with noninfectious intermediate or posterior uveitis. This was a 6-month study, one implant with no possibility of a second implant. Inclusion criteria included patients with a vitreous haze score greater than +1.5 (on a scale of 0–4) and a best corrected visual acuity (BCVA) of 20/32 to 20/630. The proportion of patients with vitreous haze score of 0 at 8 weeks was 47,

36, and 12% for the 0.7-mg DEX implant, the 0.35-mg implant, and the sham group, respectively. The response peaked at week 8 but was maintained for up to week 26. Although not used as a main outcome measure, BCVA was significantly improved 2- to 6-fold greater in the DEX-treated eyes than the sham group throughout the study period. IOP-lowering medications were required in 23% of eyes in the 0.7-mg DEX group with most patients requiring only one IOP-lowering medication. No eyes required glaucoma surgery. Cataract formation was reported in 15, 12 and 7% of DEX 0.7 mg, DEX 0.35 mg, and sham controls. One patient in the DEX 0.7 mg group required cataract surgery.

Phase IIb/III trials were carried out using the Retisert implants in uveitis, diabetic macular edema and retinal vein occlusion [37–40]. The pivotal trial in the United States randomized 278 patients with recurrent noninfectious posterior uveitis to an FA implant containing 0.59 vs. 2.1 mg. Only one eye was implanted in bilateral cases. After implantation, uveitis medications were tapered. Systemic corticosteroids were decreased by 30% per week to 2.5 mg/day for one week, then discontinued. Immunosuppressive agents were discontinued or tapered within a 6-week period at the investigator's discretion. The recurrence rate decreased in the implanted eye from 51.4% in the 34 weeks prior to implantation to 6.1% in the first 34 weeks after implantation (combined results) [24]. By comparison in the nonimplanted eye, there was an increase in the rate of recurrence from 20.3% before implantation to 42% after implantation. At 34 weeks, 51% of implanted eyes required ocular antihypertensive drops, and 5.8% underwent glaucoma filtering surgery. 10% of implanted eyes required cataract surgery. The 3-year results confirmed these initial findings with recurrence rates for the 0.59-mg implant of 4, 10, and 20% during the 1-, 2-, and 3-year postimplantation periods [39]. More implanted eyes than nonimplanted eyes had improvements in visual acuity. Mean logMAR scores were not significantly improved between baseline and year 3, but were significantly better at year 2. No improvements were observed in the control eyes. Over the 3-year follow-up, 75% of eyes required pressure-lowering medications, and 37% required IOP-lowering surgery, mainly trabeculectomies [41]. The incidence of hypotony following IOP-lowering surgery (42.5%) was not significantly different from implanted eyes not subjected to this surgery (35.4%). At 3 years, the prevalence was 11% in the 0.59-mg implant group compared to 6.1% in the fellow nonimplanted eyes. Explantations were performed for uncontrolled IOP elevation in 13 cases, over half of which required further steps to control the IOP. 93% of phakic implanted eyes underwent cataract surgery compared with only 20% of fellow phakic eyes. Most surgical procedures were carried out between week 24 and month 24 after implantation. Spontaneous dissociation of the implant from its anchoring strut was observed in a few patients leading to a redesign of the device during the course of the study [39]. A similar problem was observed on one occasion following commercialization, and may require special vitreoretinal maneuvers for removal of the dislocated implant [42, 43].

A European trial compared the 0.59-mg FA intravitreal implant to standard of care (SOC) over a 3-year period [40]. Only the worst eye was implanted. As in the pivotal trial, systemic medications were tapered but on a slower regimen over a 3-month period. Patients in the SOC group were treated according to a standardized treatment guideline. Patients receiving an implant had a significant delay in the onset of observed recurrences and overall a lower rate as compared to patients in SOC (18.2 vs. 63.5%). The incidence of glaucoma and cataract was similar to the previous study. In the implanted group, there were no treatment-related nonocular adverse events; these were observed in 26% of patients in the SOC group. Visual acuity improvements in the SOC group remained consistent over the course of the trial. In the implant group, a transient decrease at baseline was followed by a significant gain, and a further decrease between months 15 and 18, possibly related to a high incidence of cataract. By month 24, mean VA in the implanted group was similar to the screening VA, and also similar to the mean VA observed in the SOC group. Hypotony was significantly higher in the implanted eyes 19.7% compared to 1.4% of SOC study eyes. Endophthalmitis was seen in 4.5% of patients (3/66). All cases had an onset at >1 year after implant and had concomitant wound complications either at the implant site or the site of trabeculectomy. This incidence was much higher than observed in previous studies, and underscores the importance of surgical experience and meticulous wound closure.

Ocular Implants vs. Systemic Anti-Inflammatory Therapy

The MUST trial was a prospective randomized controlled parallel superiority trial initiated to compare the relative effectiveness of systemic corticosteroids plus immunosuppression vs. 0.59-mg FA intravitreal implants in noninfectious intermediate, posterior or panuveitis [44]. Participants were allocated on a 1:1 basis, with patients in the implant group receiving bilateral implant if and when required. A total of 255 patients (479 eyes) were enrolled. As in previous studies, patients receiving implants were rapidly tapered off systemic medications. Patients in the systemic treatment arm were subjected to a standardized protocol [1]. In each treatment group, mean visual acuity improved over 24 months +6.0 and +3.2 letters for the implant vs. systemic therapy group ($p = 0.16$). The results remained the same if exclusion was made of eyes better than 20/40, or when evaluating only worst eyes. Uveitis control was achieved within 9 months in both groups, but control of uveitis was more frequent in patients receiving implants (88 vs. 71% at 24 months; $p = 0.001$). The rate of improvement in vitreous haze was also more favorable. Cataract progression requiring surgery was much higher in the implanted group (80.4 vs. 31.3% cumulative 24 months) as was the incidence of increased IOP and glaucoma surgery (26.2 vs. 3.7% cumulative 24 months). In this study, the incidence of hypotony was low (8.4 vs. 6.1% cumulative 24 months). Hypertension was less frequent in implant patient ($p = 0.03$). Patients assigned to systemic therapy had more prescription-requiring infections than patients assigned to the implant therapy (0.60 vs. 0.36/person-year, $p = 0.034$). During the first 6 months, vision-related quality of life improved by 9.4 (of 100) units more than the systemic group ($p < 0.0001$); however, by 24 months both groups had improved with only a 4.6-unit advantage for the implant group. Generic health-related quality of life and health utility score were somewhat improved at the end of 24 months and favored the implant group, but the magnitude of the differences in improvement between groups was less than or equal to the threshold of previously reported minimally important differences. In their final assessment, the authors concluded that neither approach was superior over a 24-month period, particularly in view of the frequent need for additional surgery in the implant group. Specific advantages and disadvantages of either approach should guide the selection of an appropriate therapy for each individual patient. It should be noted that the low incidence of systemic side effects in patients treated systemically reflects an aggressive management approach with a rapid taper of prednisone to 10 mg or less per day and careful monitoring for systemic side effects of other immunosuppressants. The lower incidence of flare-ups in the implant group may also favor this approach after a more prolonged follow-up as recurrences are generally felt to carry a worse long-term prognosis for vision.

Treatment Paradigm in the Management of Uveitis with Steroid Implants

While the MUST trial showed that there is an equivalence in outcomes between implant and aggressive medical management with systemic medications, a number of situations can arise where the use of an ocular implant may be more appropriate than systemic therapy. The choice of implant depends on its availability, duration of action and intended use. Under no circumstances should an implant be seen as an alternative to an adequate workup and follow-up. Ruling out an infectious cause prior to the initiation of treatment cannot be overemphasized. For ophthalmologists with limited experience in uveitis, the most appropriate course of action is appropriate to refer the patient to a uveitis expert. However, the availability of implants facilitates co-management particularly in patients that must travel long distances. In each of the scenarios described below, you should consider whether you are dealing with unilateral or bilateral disease, whether uveitis is symmetrical or asymmetrical, and the expected duration of inflammation.

Uveitis with Systemic Disease

In patients with systemic disease requiring high doses of steroids or immunosuppression with bilateral uveitis requiring treatment, the most judicious course of action would call for an adjustment in systemic immunomodulation (fig. 1). In this

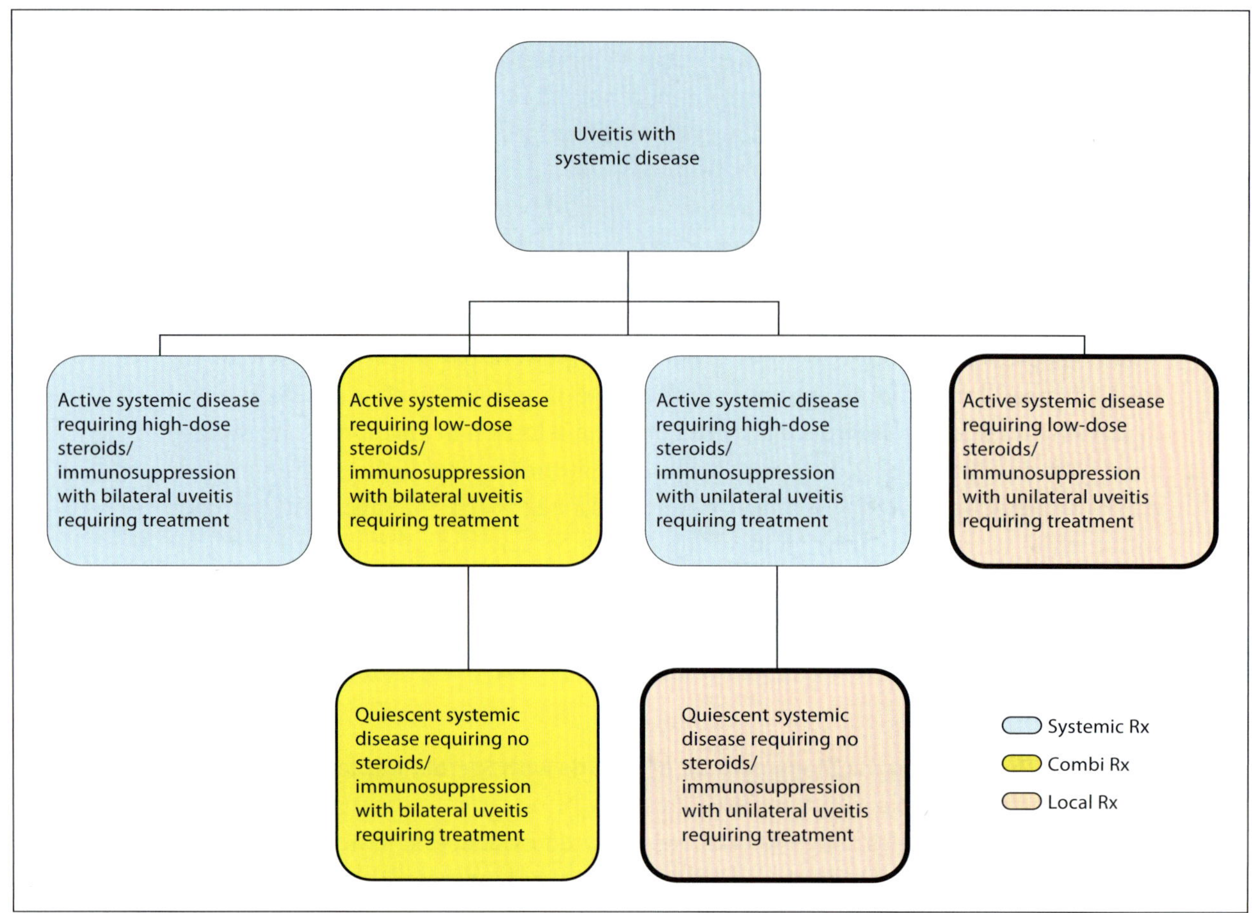

Fig. 1. Proposed treatment algorithm for the treatment of uveitis patients with a systemic autoimmune disease.

particular situation, management is most often carried out in conjunction with an internist or rheumatologist. A similar approach should be considered in patients with active systemic disease and unilateral uveitis requiring treatment. In the presence of bilateral active uveitis, but where the systemic disease requires only low doses of steroids/immunosuppression or is quiescent not requiring immunosuppression, the treatment of choice for the eyes could involve an increase in systemic therapy to calm the less severe of the two eyes, while implanting the more affected eye. This approach has the advantage of titrating immunomodulation based on the observed inflammatory response in an attempt to minimize both systemic and local side effects. Presence of ocular inflammation is a sign of persistent systemic activity which may require some degree of systemic immunosuppression but is likely to be much less than that required to control the ocular disease. In cases of unilateral ocular inflammation, it is clear that the most appropriate course of action will be the use of an intraocular implant with close follow-up of the noninvolved eye.

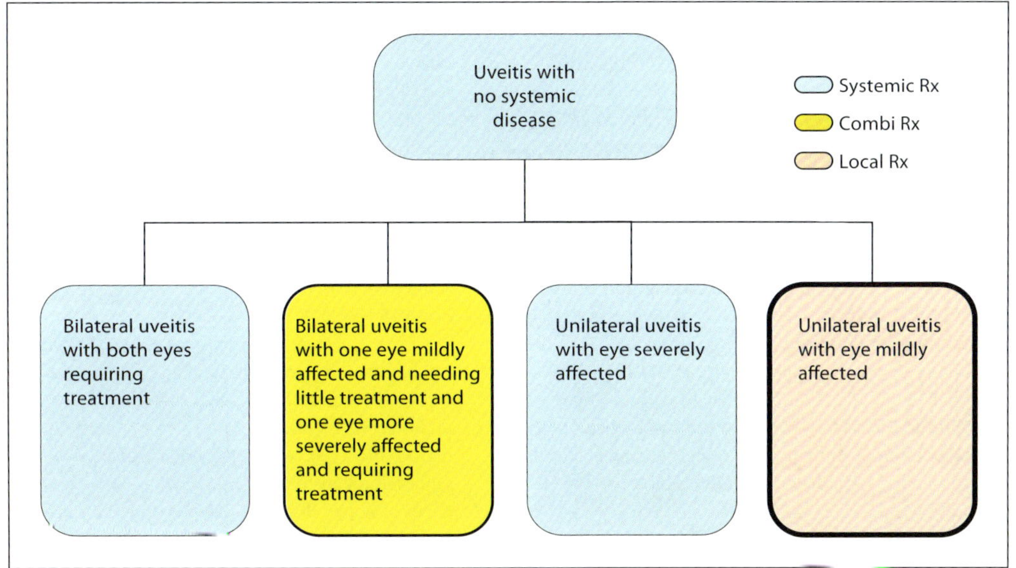

Fig. 2. Proposed treatment algorithm for the treatment of uveitis patients with no systemic autoimmune disease.

Uveitis with No Systemic Disease

Systemic therapy should be considered in cases of bilateral severe uveitis or when one eye is severely affected (fig. 2). It is likely in this scenario that systemic treatment will be aimed at a rapid reduction of inflammation by for example the use of pulsed methylprednisolone, high-dose steroids with or without the adjunct of nonsteroidal immunosuppressants. Once the inflammation is brought under control, long-term management may involve the use of an implant in one or both eyes. The aim in this case is to minimize exposure to systemic immunosuppression while providing high level immunosuppression to the eye. In cases of unilateral uveitis of moderate severity, implantation could be considered immediately.

Specific Medical Conditions

Patients intolerant to systemic steroids, with a history of diabetes, gastrointestinal tract ulceration, osteoporosis, hypertension or pregnancy even in the presence of bilateral disease may be more appropriately treated with a steroid implant. Similarly, patients requiring ocular surgery with a prior history of uveitis or with controlled uveitis on systemic immunosuppression may benefit from an implant placed at the time of surgery. Depending on the degree and type of ocular inflammation, the use of an implant may obviate the need for presurgical systemic immunosuppression.

References

1 Jabs DA, Rosenbaum JT, Foster CS, Holland GN, Jaffe GJ, Louie JS, Nussenblatt RB, Stiehm ER, Tessler H, Van Gelder RN, Whitcup SM, Yocum D: Guidelines for the use of immunosuppressive drugs in patients with ocular inflammatory disorders: recommendations of an expert panel. Am J Ophthalmol 2000;130:492–513.

2 Nguyen QD, Hatef E, Kayen B, Macahilig CP, Ibrahim M, Wang J, Shaikh O, Bodaghi B: A cross-sectional study of the current treatment patterns in noninfectious uveitis among specialists in the United States. Ophthalmology 2011;118:184–190.

3 Shen L, You Y, Sun S, Chen Y, Qu J, Cheng L: Intraocular and systemic pharmacokinetics of triamcinolone acetonide after a single 40-mg posterior subtenon application. Ophthalmology 2010;117: 2365–2371.

4 Venkatesh P, Kumar CS, Abbas Z, Garg S: Comparison of the efficacy and safety of different methods of posterior subtenon injection. Ocul Immunol Inflamm 2008;16:217–223.

5 Rhen T, Cidlowski JA: Antiinflammatory action of glucocorticoids – new mechanisms for old drugs. New Engl J Med 2005;353:1711–1723.

6 de Bosscher K, Vanden Berghe W, Haegeman G: The interplay between the glucocorticoid receptor and nuclear factor-κb or activator protein-1: molecular mechanisms for gene repression. Endoc Rev 2003;24:488–522.

7 Edelman JL: Differentiating intraocular glucocorticoids. Ophthalmologica 2010;224:25–30.

8 McKenzie AW, Stoughton RB: Method for comparing percutaneous absorption of steroids. Arch Dermatol 1962;86:608–610.

9 Kelly HW: Pharmaceutical characteristics that influence the clinical efficacy of inhaled corticosteroids. Ann Allerg Asthma Immunol 2003;91:326–334.

10 Nehme A, Lobenhofer E, Stamer WD, Edelman J: Glucocorticoids with different chemical structures but similar glucocorticoid receptor potency regulate subsets of common and unique genes in human trabecular meshwork cells. BMC Med Genomics 2009; 2:58.

11 Fan BJ, Wang DY, Tham CC, Lam DS, Pang CP: Gene expression profiles of human trabecular meshwork cells induced by triamcinolone and dexamethasone. Invest Ophthalmol Vis Sci 2008;49:1886–1897.

12 Wenzel A, Grimm C, Seeliger MW, Jaissle G, Hafezi F, Kretschmer R, Zrenner E, Remé CE: Prevention of photoreceptor apoptosis by activation of the glucocorticoid receptor. Invest Ophthalmol Vis Sci 2001;42:1653–1659.

13 Glybina IV, Kennedy A, Ashton P, Abrams GW, Iezzi R: Photoreceptor neuroprotection in RCS rats via low-dose intravitreal sustained-delivery of fluocinolone acetonide. Invest Ophthalmol Vis Sci 2009; 50:4847–4857.

14 Valamanesh F, Berdugo M, Sennlaub F, Savoldelli M, Goumeaux C, Houssier M, Jeanny JC, Torriglia A, Behar-Cohen F: Effects of triamcinolone acetonide on vessels of the posterior segment of the eye. Mol Vis 2009;15:2634–2648.

15 Torriglia A, Valamanesh F, Behar-Cohen F: On the retinal toxicity of intraocular glucocorticoids. Biochem Pharm 2010;80:1878–1886.

16 de Smet MD, Julian K: The role of steroids in the management of uveitic macular edema. Eur J Ophthalmol 2011;21:51–55.

17 Chang-Lin J-E, Burke JA, Peng Q, Lin T, Orilla WC, Ghosn CR, Zhang K-M, Kuppermann BD, Robinson MR, Whitcup SM, Welty DF: Pharmacokinetics of a sustained-release dexamethasone intravitreal implant in vitrectomized and nonvitrectomized eyes. Invest Ophthalmol Vis Sci 2011;52:4605–4609.

18 Chang-Lin JE, Attar M, Acheampong AA, Robinson MR, Whitcup SM, Kuppermann BD, Welty D: Pharmacokinetics and pharmacodynamics of the sustained-release dexamethasone intravitreal implant. Invest Ophthalmol Vis Sci 2011;52:80–86.

19 Schindler RH, Chandler DB, Thresker R, Machemer R: The clearance of intravitreal triamcinolone acetonide. Am J Ophthalmol 1982;93:415–417.

20 Lee S, Ghosn C, Yu Z, Zacharias LC, Kao H, Lanni C, Abdelfattah N, Juppermann B, Csaky KG, D'Argenio DZ, Burke JA, Hughes PM, Robinson MR: Vitreous VEGF clearance is increased after vitrectomy. Invest Ophthalmol Vis Sci 2010;51: 2135–2138.

21 Doft B, Weiskopf J, Nilsson-Ehle I, Wingard L Jr: Amphotericin clearance in vitrectomized versus nonvitrectomized eyes. Ophthalmology 1985;92: 1601–1605.

22 Jaffe GJ, Ben-nun J, Guo H, Dunn JP, Ashton P: Fluocinolone acetonide sustained drug delivery device to treat severe uveitis. Ophthalmology 2000; 107:2024–2033.

23 Driot JY, Novack GD, Rittenhouse KD, Milazzo C, Pearson PA: Ocular pharmacokinetics of fluocinolone acetonide after Retisert intravitreal implantation in rabbits over a 1-year period. J Ocul Pharm Ther 2004;20:269–275.

24 Jaffe GJ, Martin D, Callanan D, Pearson PA, Levy B, Comstock T: Fluocinolone acetonide implant (Retisert) for noninfectious posterior uveitis: thirty-four-week results of a multicenter randomized clinical study. Ophthalmology 2006;113:1020–1027.

25 Perkins SL, Gallemore RP, Yang CH, Guo H, Ashton P, Jaffe GJ: Pharmacokinetics of the fluocinolone/5-fluorouracil codrug in the gas-filled eye. Retina 2000;20:514–519.

26 Kane FE, Burdan J, Cutino A, Green KE: Iluvien: a new sustained delivery technology for posterior eye disease. Expert Opin Drug Deliv 2006;5:1039–1046.

27 Campochiaro PA, Hafiz G, Shah SM, Bloom S, Brown DM, Busquets M, Ciulla T, Feiner L, Sabates N, Billman K, Kapik B, Green K, Kane F: Sustained ocular delivery of fluocinolone acetonide by an intravitreal insert. Ophthalmology 2010;117:1393–1399, e1393.

28 Kim H, Robinson MR, Lizak MJ, Tansey G, Lutz RJ, Yuan P, Wang NS, Csaky KG: Controlled drug release from an ocular implant: an evaluation using dynamic three-dimensional magnetic resonance imaging. Invest Ophthalmol Vis Sci 2004;45:2722–2731.

29 Li SK, Lizak MJ, Jeong EK: MRI in ocular drug delivery. NMR Biomed 2008;21:941–956.

30 Thakur A, Kadam R, Kompella UB: Trabecular meshwork and lens partitioning of corticosteroids: implications for elevated intraocular pressure and cataracts. Archiv Ophthalmol 2011;129:914–920.

31 James ER: The etiology of steroid cataract. J Ocul Pharmacol Ther 2007;23:403–420.

32 Szabó V, Borgulya G, Filkorn T, Majnik J, Bányász I, Nagy ZZ: The variant n363s of glucocorticoid receptor in steroid-induced ocular hypertension in Hungarian patients treated with photorefractive keratectomy. Mol Vis 2007;13:659–666.

33 Haller JA, Bandello F, Belfort R Jr, Blumenkranz MS, Gillies M, Heier J, Loewenstein A, Yoon Y-H, Jacques M-L, Jiao J, Li X-Y, Whitcup SM: Randomized, sham-controlled trial of dexamethasone intravitreal implant in patients with macular edema due to retinal vein occlusion. Ophthalmology 2010;117:1134–1146, e1133.

34 Boyer DS, Faber DJ, Gupta SK, Patel SS, Tabandeh H, Li XY, Liu CC, Lou J, Whitcup SM, for the Ozurdex Champlain Study Group: Dexamethasone intravitreal implant for treatment of diabetic macular edema in vitrectomized patients. Retina 2011;31:915–923.

35 Lowder C, Belfort R Jr, Lightman S, Foster CS, Robinson MR, Schiffman RM, Li X-Y, Cui H, Whitcup SM, for the Ozurdex HSG: Dexamethasone intravitreal implant for noninfectious intermediate or posterior uveitis. Arch Ophthalmol 2011;129:545–553.

36 London NJ, Chiang A, Haller JA: The dexamethasone drug delivery system: indications and evidence. Adv Ther 2011;28:351–366.

37 Pearson PA, Comstock TL, Ip MS, Callanan D, Morse LS, Ashton P, Levy B, Mann ES, Eliott D: Fluocinolone acetonide intravitreal implant for diabetic macular edema: a 3-year multicenter, randomized, controlled clinical trial. Ophthalmology 2011;118:1580–1586.

38 Jain N, Stinnett SS, Jaffe GJ: Prospective study of a fluocinolone acetonide implant for chronic macular edema from central retinal vein occlusion thirty-six-month results. Ophthalmology 2012;119:132–137.

39 Callanan DG, Jaffe GJ, Martin DF, Pearson PA, Comstock TL: Treatment of posterior uveitis with a fluocinolone acetonide implant: three-year clinical trial results. Arch Ophthalmol 2008;126:1191–1201.

40 Pavesio C, Zierhut M, Bairi K, Comstock TL, Usner DW: Evaluation of an intravitreal fluocinolone acetonide implant versus standard systemic therapy in noninfectious posterior uveitis. Ophthalmology 2010;117:567–575.

41 Goldstein DA, Godfrey DG, Hall AJH, Callanan DG, Jaffe GJ, Pearson A, Usner DW, Comstock TL: Intraocular pressure in patients with uveitis treated with fluocinolone acetonide implants. Arch Ophthalmol 2007;125:1478–1485.

42 Yeh S, Cebulla DM, Witherspoon SR, Emerson GG, Emerson MV, Suhler EB, Albini TA, Flaxel CJ: Management of fluocinolone implant dissociation during implant exchange. Arch Ophthalmol 2009;127:1218–1221.

43 Wan W, Stewart JM: Use of a high infusion rate to prevent posterior dislocation of fluocinolone acetonide implant during surgical removal. Ocul Immunol Inflamm 2011;19:214–215.

44 Multicenter Uveitis Steroid Treatment (MUST) Trial Research Group, Kempen JH, Altaweel MM, Holbrook JT, Jabs DA, Louis TA, Sugar EA, Thorne JE: Randomized comparison of systemic anti-inflammatory therapy versus fluocinolone acetonide implant for intermediate, posterior, and panuveitis: the multicenter uveitis steroid treatment trial. Ophthalmology 2011;118:1916–1926.

Marc D. de Smet
Chemin des Allinges 10
CH–1001 Lausanne (Switzerland)
Tel. +41 21 619 3858, E-Mail mddesmet1@mac.com

Miserocchi E, Modorati G, Foster CS (eds): New Treatments in Noninfectious Uveitis.
Dev Ophthalmol. Basel, Karger, 2012, vol 51, pp 134–161

New Treatment Options for Noninfectious Uveitis

Millena Gomes Bittencourt · Yasir Jamal Sepah · Diana V. Do · Owhofasa Agbedia · Abeer Akhtar · Hongting Liu · Anam Akhlaq · Rachel Annam · Mohamed Ibrahim · Quan Dong Nguyen

Retinal Imaging Research and Reading Center, Wilmer Eye Institute, Johns Hopkins University, Baltimore, Md., USA

Abstract

Autoimmune uveitis is a group of sight-threatening inflammatory diseases associated with an exacerbated immunological response to ocular proteins. The Standardization of Uveitis Nomenclature Working Group Guidelines have recommended the use of corticosteroids as the first line of therapy for patients who present with active uveitis. However, long-term use of corticosteroids is associated with numerous adverse effects including cataract, glaucoma and metabolic disorders. In this context, new drugs developed to treat rheumatic diseases, and other autoimmune diseases, are being employed often as monotherapy or combined with other immunosuppressive drugs in order to decrease the corticosteroid burden on patients and to manage refractive uveitis. These drugs are currently being evaluated in the framework of uveitis and may open a new horizon with less side effects and more responsiveness for chronic cases. Among others, calcineurin inhibitor voclosporin, mammalian target of rapamycin inhibitor sirolimus, and the IL-1 trap rilonacept, are among these new agents and will be scrutinized in detail in this chapter. More efficient modes of drug delivery are also being employed to deliver high concentration of drug locally and to minimize systemic side effects. The new modes of drug delivery that we will describe in the index chapter include nanoparticles and iontophoresis.

Uveitis encompasses a group of potentially blinding inflammatory diseases. The Standardization of Uveitis Nomenclature (SUN) Working Group classifies uveitis according to the anatomic location of disease [1]. Anterior uveitis can involve the cornea, iris, and/or anterior ciliary body. Intermediate uveitis affects the middle structures of the eye, such as the posterior ciliary body. Posterior uveitis can involve the vitreous, choroid, retina, and/or optic nerve. Panuveitis, also referred to as diffuse, can encompass anterior, intermediate, and posterior segments [1]. Anterior uveitis is the most common location, constituting 60–75% of the cases and being chronic in up to two-thirds of the patients [2, 3]. Conversely, posterior uveitis is usually associated with more frequent irreversible visual impairment and is more challenging to manage. The importance of this sight-threatening disease is translated in numbers. Studies have estimated that uveitis may lead to legal blindness in 30,000 patients annually [4, 5]. It is estimated that uveitis is the cause of 2.8–10% of all cases of blindness, and the annual cost associated with the disease in the United States alone hovers around USD 242.6 million [6, 7]. In the United States, uveitis has an incidence of 25–52 cases per 100,000 persons per year, although some studies have shown that it can vary worldwide, from 38 to 730 cases per 100,000 persons per year [4, 8, 9].

Pathogenesis

Understanding the pathogenesis of uveitis is complicated by the fact that it encompasses a wide range of underlying etiologies. The inflammation present in uveitis can be triggered by an infectious agent, a traumatic insult to the eye, or by an imbalance between the ocular immune privilege and an autoimmune response. The noninfectious uveitis of a putative autoimmune nature, also known as endogenous uveitis, affects patients of different age groups, and can be limited to the eye or be part of a systemic syndrome. The autoimmune causality is supported by strong human leukocyte antigen (HLA) association and by the demonstration of errant responses to retinal antigens in animals models [10, 11]. Two principal models have been used to study autoimmune uveitis: the endotoxin-induced uveitis (EIU), representing a nonspecific, innate efferent immune response (inflammation), and the experimental autoimmune uveitis (EAU), which includes the afferent arm (antigen-specific activation of T cells) and the subsequent ocular inflammation [12]. These two models have shown that during the effector phase of uveitis, humoral and cellular components of the immune system trigger a cascade of events that ultimately lead to tissue destruction. The cells involved in EIU are monocytes/macrophages and polymorphonuclear neutrophils, the key players of inflammation. Thereafter, the tumor necrosis factor-α (TNF-α) cytokine is essential for the induction of EIU, and along with the interleukin (IL)-6 produced in the eye, plays a major role in the development of ocular inflammation [13, 14]. Two different types of T helper cells, the Th1 type and/or the Th17 type, are able to drive the ocular autoimmune activity, as demonstrated by the EAU model [15] (fig. 1). The Th1 response has been related to R14-specific T cell and with more relapsing disease than seen in the Th17 response [16]. During the autoimmune activity, T cells release cytokines including various ILs (IL-1, IL-2, IL-4, IL-6, IL-17, IL-21 and IL-22) [17], interferon-γ (INF-γ) and TNF-α that work as signaling molecules towards the amplification and sustenance of the inflammatory process [18–20]. IL-10 is also involved in the autoimmune process and the increase in IL-10 mRNA expression in late disease may reflect its role in the disease resolution [18]. Complement also plays an important role in the induction of antigen-specific T cell responses in EAU. Complement activation products such as C3b and C4b

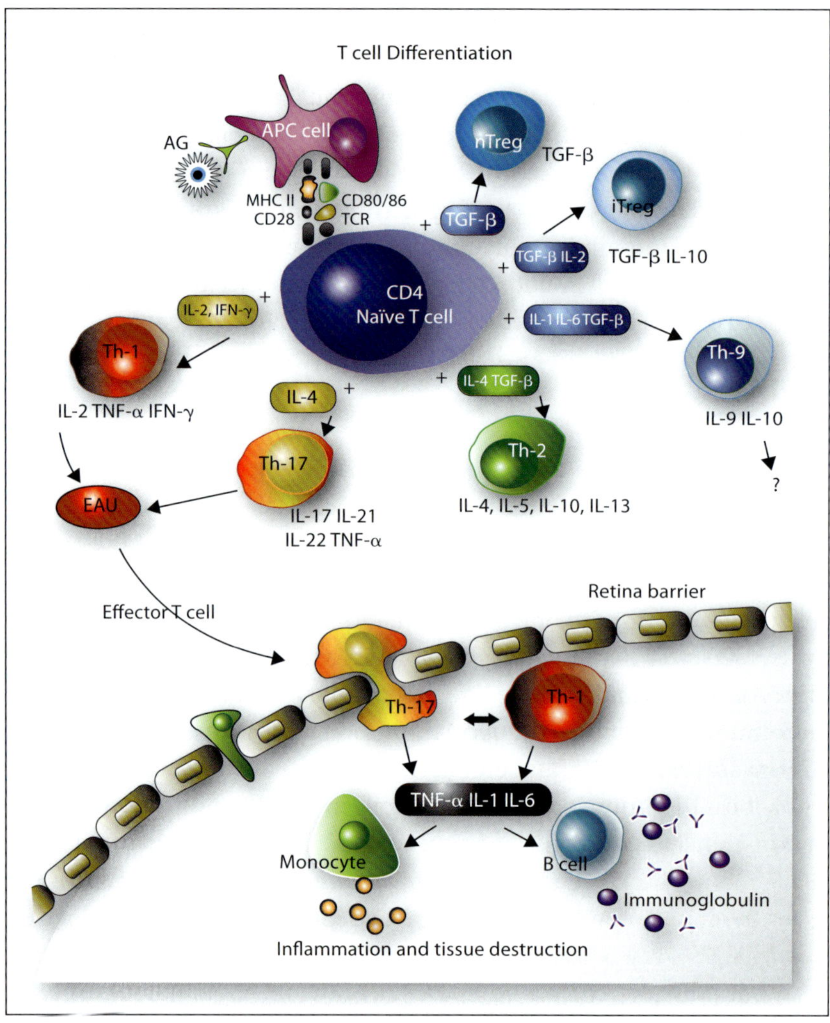

Fig. 1. Illustrative scheme of the CD4 T cell activation by antigen-presenting cells (APCs), differentiation and recruitment to the chorioretinal tissue. The cytokine network associated with uveitis is illustrated based on currently available information from the literature and role(s) of each subset in the animal models of EAU. The naïve CD4 T cells recognize a complex of class II MHC and peptide present on the surface of APCs. This results in signaling via the T cell receptor (TCR) which combined with a specific cytokine profile leads to a specific Th cell subset differentiation (Th1, Th17, Th2, Th9 and Tregs). TCR engagement in the absence of costimulatory (CD28) signals is thought to produce tolerance by inducing nonresponsiveness to specific antigens and promoting apoptotic deletion of the activated cells (activation-induced cell death). AG = Antigen.

have been demonstrated to increase during the active phase of the disease [21]. Major histocompatibility complex (MHC class I and II) and adhesion molecules (ICAM-1 and LECAM-1) are some other molecules upregulated by the cytokine release, facilitating the migration of leukocytes to the inflamed eye and contributing to the inflammatory cascade, consequently leading to a chronic uveitis [22–24].

The rationale of targeting the etiologic agent of any pathology is the ideal way to stop its progression and sequelae. However, this rationale is not applicable to uveitis. The etiologic triggers of the vigorous immunologic and inflammatory responses against ocular antigens are poorly understood, and the mechanism by which the immune privilege is lost is yet to be described. Thus, targeting the inflammatory pathway is the only available way to manage this sight-threatening disease and to avoid further sequels as cataract, glaucoma, proliferative vitreoretinopathy, cystoid macular edema (CME), vascular occlusion and blindness [25]. A better understanding of the immunologic process in the last few decades has made possible the identification of key points in the inflammatory chain that can be targeted to stop the pathology. These potential targets are described in table 1.

Standard Therapies

Since its first use in 1951, corticosteroids remain as the first line therapy in the armamentarium against uveitis. This is the only class of drug approved by the United States Food and Drug Administration (FDA) to treat uveitis and ocular inflammatory diseases [26]. Different routes of administration and different formulations are available. Topical corticosteroids penetrate well only into the anterior chamber of the eye, and are useful in the management of anterior uveitis and episcleritis. Periocular injections of steroids offer the benefit of a local high-dose and great penetration into the posterior segment, making them a good choice to treat intermediate uveitis, CME and posterior uveitis [27]. Intravitreal (ITV) injection provides the most direct route to posterior segment, thus potentially greater efficacy for posterior uveitis and CME than oral or periocular injection. However, ITV delivery of steroid is also most likely to be associated with ocular side effects, including cataract, high intraocular pressure and endophthalmitis [28]. Steroid implants have the benefit of sustained corticosteroid delivery to the eye while avoiding complications of systemic therapy. Fluocinolone acetonide and dexamethasone are the two corticosteroid compounds in the FDA-approved intraocular implants Retisert® and Ozurdex®, respectively. A multicenter randomized clinical trial comparing 0.59- to 2.1-mg fluocinolone acetonide implant for uveitis has shown improvement and stabilization of visual acuity in patients with noninfectious uveitis. No significant difference in mean LogMAR VA at the 1- or 3-year postimplantation visit compared to the baseline for either the 0.59-mg group or the 2.1-mg group was observed. However, there was a significant improvement in LogMAR VA at the 2-year postimplantation visit for both dose groups and a deterioration in mean LogMAR VA in fellow nonimplanted eyes at all 3 postimplantation visits ($p < 0.01$). The one-year postimplantation recurrence rates in the 0.59 mg group dropped from 62 to 4%, and in the 2.1 mg group from 58 to 7% in 3 years. During the course of the 3-year study, 78% (both groups combined) of the patients required intraocular pressure-lowering drops, 40% required glaucoma surgery and 93% of eyes required cataract extraction. While the frequency of IOP-

Table 1. Potential immune targets

Target	Class	Role in EAU	Clinical relevance
Cytokines	IFN-γ	This proinflammatory cytokine is essential for the induction of Th1 lineage. The early production of IFN-γ in the EAU has a paradoxical protective effect.	Elevated in AqH, aqueous humor of BD, VKH
	TNF-α	This proinflammatory cytokine is involved in systemic inflammation and is a member of a group of cytokines that stimulate the acute phase reaction.	Elevated serum level in BD
Interleukins	Th1 lineage: IL-12	This is the major pathogenic effector T cell subset in uveitis. The IL-12 is the key Th1-inducing cytokine, and IL-2 and IFN-γ are the molecules released by this subset of T cells.	Elevated in BD
	IL-2	This cytokine stimulates the growth, differentiation and survival of antigen-selected cytotoxic T cells via the activation of the expression of specific genes.	Elevated in serum and AqH in uveitis
	Th2 and Th9 lineage: IL-4, IL-10, IL-13, and IL-9	Th2: The suppressive cell subset, also known as Treg cells, could be ascribed to their IL-10 production.	Increased levels were paradoxically found in the serum of BD
		Th9: This cell subset can be induced in presence of IL-4 and produces IL-9 and IL-10. The role of the IL-9 and of the Th9 in uveitis requires further investigation.	N/A
	Th17 lineage: IL-17A, IL-17F, IL-21, IL-22, and IL-23.	This proinflammatory cell subset is stimulated by IL-23 and produces IL-17. This IL acts as a potent mediator in delayed-type reactions by increasing chemokine production in various tissues to recruit monocytes and neutrophils to the site of inflammation, similar to IFN-γ.	Increased expression in PBMC and serum of BD, VKH
	IL-6	IL-6 has been shown to be a critical mediator for induction of inflammation and for Th17 differentiation.	Increased in the serum, AqH and vitreous.
	TGF-β, IL-10, IL-27, and IL-35	This profile has been shown to have suppressive activity in autoimmune diseases. However, TGF-β was recently identified as a critical cytokine for Th17 and Th9 differentiation when acting in concert with other cytokines (IL-1b or IL-6 for Th17 and IL-4 for Th9).	Decreased level in AqH.

Table 1. Continued

Target	Class	Role in EAU	Clinical relevance
Adhesion molecules	ICAM-1	Neutrophil migration through blood vessels into inflamed tissues.	Evidence in Crohn's disease.
	VCAM-1	It is expressed on the surface of activated endothelial cells, dendritic cells, fibroblasts, and tissue macrophages, and facilitates entry of activated leukocytes through blood vessels into inflamed tissues.	High levels in iris biopsy specimens from patients with anterior uveitis.
Receptors	CTLA-4	In addition to T cell receptor recognition of the peptide/MHC complex on antigen-presenting cells, costimulatory signals are needed to fully activate a naive T cell. Those costimulatory signals are mediated by CD28 binding to CD80 or CD86 on the surface of T cells and on APC. Upon TCR ligation, CTLA-4 or CD152, another ligand of CD80/CD86 is upregulated on the surface of T helper cells.	N/A
	CD-20	The surface antigen CD20 is expressed on pre-B and mature B cells. Important in the secretion of proinflammatory cytokines, antigen presentation, T cell activation, and autoantibody production.	N/A
	CD-52	CD-52 is a glycoprotein expressed on the surface of all mature lymphocytes and also found on dendritic cells and monocytes. Its precise function is still unknown.	N/A

AqH = Aqueous humor; BD = Behçet's disease; VKH = Vogt-Koyanagi-Harada disease; N/A = information not available; IFN-γ = interferon-γ; DC = dendritic cells; PBMC = peripheral blood mononuclear cells; TGF-β = transforming growth factor-β; Treg cells = regulatory T cells; ICAM-1 = intercellular adhesion molecule 1; VCAM = vascular cell adhesion molecule, CD-20 = cluster of differentiation 20; CD-58 = cluster of differentiation 58.

lowering surgery began to increase by postimplantation week 12 for implanted eyes, most of the cataract extraction procedures performed occurred between postimplantation week 24 and month 24 [29, 30]. Vitreous band formation, and very rarely endophthalmitis, has also been reported after ITV implant [28].

The systemic usage of corticosteroid is often the choice to treat bilateral disease, anterior uveitis associated with CME, and those with sight-threatening posterior uveitis. However, a great number of patients cannot tolerate its dose-dependent side effects. Cushingoid syndrome, diabetes, osteoporotic bones, and metabolic disturbances are the most common side effects [26, 34]. Treatment guidelines were developed by an expert panel and reinforced by the SUN Working Group [27]. To decrease the risk of serious side effects associated with systemic long-term corticosteroid use, guidelines recommend the addition of immunomodulatory therapy (IMT) as a steroid-sparing agent if inflammation cannot be controlled with ≤10 mg/day of prednisone (or equivalent) within 3 months [1]. However, not all types of uveitis will respond to steroids. Recently, a study from the UK has demonstrated the existence of a subpopulation of CD4+ cell refractive to dexamethasone therapy [32] in patients with refractory uveitis.

IMT may not only serve as a good alternative to control the inflammatory process but also to reduce the corticosteroid side effects. While corticosteroids are usually required to control acute inflammation, IMT agents are often needed to downregulate chronic inflammation and prevent recurrences. The majority of IMT agents take several weeks to achieve therapeutic tissue levels; hence, initially, these agents are typically administered in combination with oral corticosteroids to control acute inflammation. Once the disease is quiet, the corticosteroids are tapered or, if possible, discontinued [27]. IMT agents can be categorized into 3 main classes: the T cell inhibitors (cyclosporine and tacrolimus), the antimetabolites (azathioprine, methotrexate, mycophenolate mofetil and leflunomide), and the alkylating agents (cyclophosphamide and chlorambucil). The antimetabolites have their therapeutic effects by interfering with nucleic acid synthesis required for DNA replication and cell proliferation [28]. The alkylating agents have their effect by covalently modifying DNA. Drugs like cyclosporine target primarily T cells and have demonstrated efficacy when employed in the treatment of uveitis [27, 35]. Systemic cyclosporine has been approved in Germany and in a few other countries for treatment of refractory uveitis, but has not been approved in the United States. Tacrolimus, another IMT agent closely related to cyclosporine, has shown effectiveness in uveitis refractory to cyclosporine in previous studies [36, 37]. Bone marrow suppression, neurotoxicity, nephrotoxicity, hepatitis, pneumonitis, diarrhea and infertility are some of the possible and not uncommon adverse effects of immunosuppressants [38]. A cohort study named SITE (Methods for Identifying Long-Term Adverse Effects of Treatment in Patients with Eye Diseases: The Systemic Immunosuppressive Therapy for Eye Diseases Cohort Study) was conducted in the US to identify the long-term adverse events of IMT in patients with uveitis. The study demonstrated that alkylating agents followed by azathioprine, cyclosporine, and methotrexate, respectively, increases the risks of fatal malignancy and mortality when compared with normal population [33, 38]. These serious side effects are the main reason that treatment must be individualized and regularly monitored [27].

New Agents in the Uveitis Pharmacotherapy: Emerging Drugs

An increasing number of new drugs based on immunomodulation and immunosuppression have been evaluated in clinical trials during the last few years. Less toxicity, more effectiveness, ability to rescue refractory cases, corticosteroid-sparing benefits, and action in different targets in the inflammatory pathways are the ideal characteristics of a new drug. New drugs derived from agents already used to treat autoimmune diseases are currently in clinical evaluation for uveitis, including the new generation of calcineurin inhibitors. More recently, biologic agents have been explored for use in uveitis, including TNF-α inhibitors (infliximab, etanercept, and adalimumab), anti-lymphocyte agents (rituximab and alemtuzumab), and an IL-2 receptor blocker (daclizumab) [39]. Potentially new therapeutic agents can be defined as treatments that employ an agonist or an antagonist to enhance specifically or to suppress the level of a naturally occurring protein molecule to manipulate a disease state [39], and can get the effect directly against the signal molecules or their receptors [40].

Inhibitors of T Cell Activation

New Generation of the Calcineurin Inhibitors: Voclosporin

Voclosporin (E-ISA247) is a next-generation calcineurin inhibitor that originated from a modification of a functional group on the first amino acid residue of the cyclosporin A (CsA) molecule [31]. Voclosporin reversibly inhibits T cell proliferation, prevents release of proinflammatory cytokines, fibroblast proliferation and vascular endothelial growth factor (VEGF) expression [41–44]. After entering the lymphocyte cytoplasm, calcineurin inhibitors bind to immunophilins and form complexes that subsequently bind to and inhibit calcineurin, a calcium-regulated enzyme, also known as serine-threonine phosphatase calcineurin [44, 45]. This process prevents translocation of the cytoplasmic component of the nuclear factor of activated T cells to the nucleus, which in turn impairs transcription of the genes encoding IL-2 and other lymphokines [42, 44] (fig. 2). In vitro studies have shown that voclosporin is approximately four times more potent than CsA, and is therefore likely to have an improved safety profile as lower therapeutic doses can be used. The higher activity of voclosporin can be explained by superior Van der Waals interactions between its unique side chain and cyclophilin A [46].

Voclosporin is currently being employed for the treatment of psoriasis and organ transplant rejection (Isotechnika Inc., 2008). The drug has been evaluated in 3 phase III studies to support clinical development for noninfectious uveitis.

Evaluation of Voclosporin Efficacy

The LUMINATE (LX211 Uveitis Multicenter Investigation of a New Approach to TrEatment) studies evaluated the efficacy of voclosporin for noninfectious uveitis in three placebo-controlled, dose-ranging, randomized, multicenter trials (The LUMINATE Active, the LUMINATE Maintenance, and the LUMINATE Anterior) [47]. The studies included a broad spectrum of subjects with a variety of etiologies of uveitis involving the anterior, intermediate, and/or posterior segments and disease status (active and quiescent) that required systemic IMT with or without systemic corticosteroids. Two hundred and eighteen patients were enrolled in this study at 57 centers

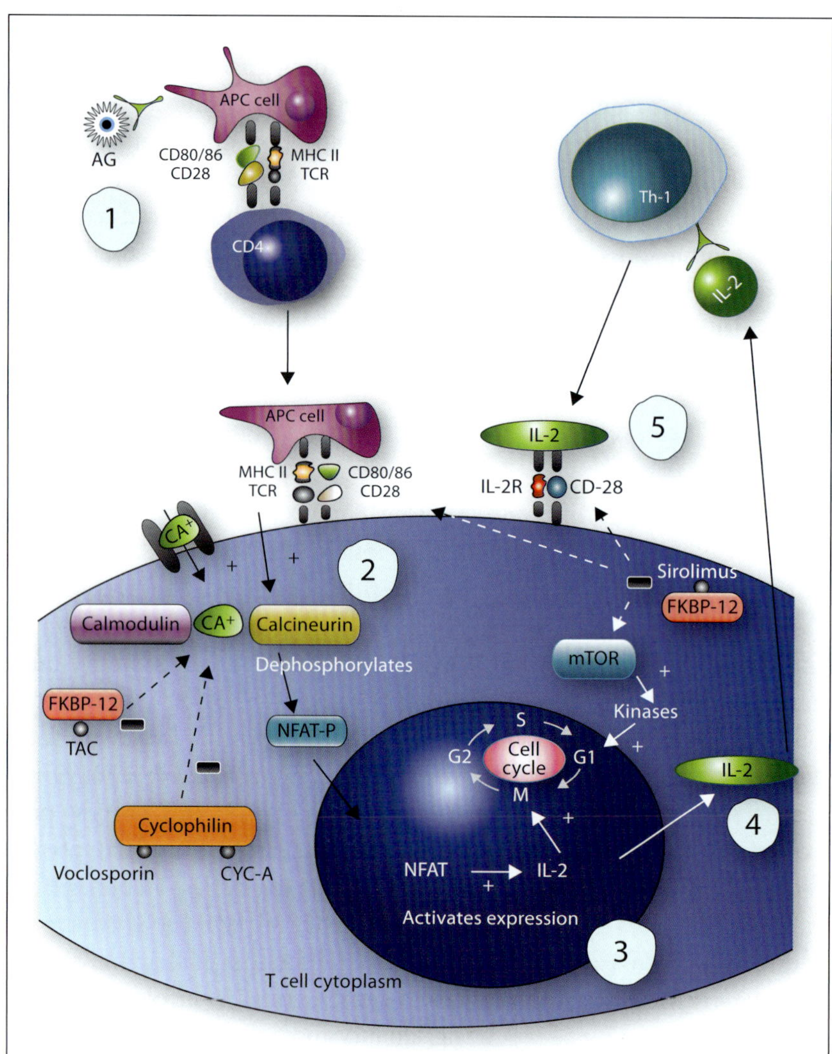

Fig. 2. Mechanism of action of the T cell inhibitors and sirolimus. CD4-positive T cells recognize a complex of class II MHC and peptide present on the surface of APCs (1). This results in signaling via the TCR and activation of calcineurin, a phosphatase (3). Calcineurin dephosphorylates NFAT (nuclear factor of activated T cells) facilitating its transfer into the nucleus, where it acts as a transcription factor regulating IL-2 production (4). IL-2 and other cytokines in turn promote further T cell activation and proliferation following interaction with its cell surface receptor (IL-2R; 5). Of note, TCR engagement alone is insufficient to produce an immune response. Costimulatory signals (via CD28) are also necessary to produce and sustain a T cell response. TCR engagement in the absence of costimulatory signals is thought to produce tolerance by inducing nonresponsiveness to specific antigens and promoting apoptotic deletion of the activated cells (activation-induced cell death). Cyclosporin and tacrolimus (FK506) act by binding to their respective immunophilins (cyclophilin/FK-binding protein, FKBP-12) with the resultant complexes producing calcineurin inhibition (black-dash arrows). The net effect is blockade of IL-2 production, resulting in inhibition of T cell activation. Sirolimus also binds the same cytosolic receptor – FKBP-12. However, in this case, the complex binds the mTOR, resulting in disruption of IL-2 receptor signaling and inhibition of T cell proliferation (by inducing cell cycle arrest). Sirolimus also blocks costimulatory signals generated by the engagement of CD28, which may be beneficial in inducing tolerance (white-dash arrows).

in America, Europe, and India. The studies compared three dosages of voclosporin: 0.2, 0.4, and 0.6 mg/kg b.i.d. with placebo in patients with different types of uveitis [47, 48].

In the LX211-01 (Treatment of Active Intermediate and Posterior Uveitis, and Panuveitis) study, voclosporin has demonstrated a rapid onset of action either alone or in combination with systemic corticosteroids. The drug also reduced inflammation in moderately severe disease, as evidenced by the improvement of the vitreous haze. Subjects receiving voclosporin 0.4 mg/kg b.i.d. experienced a 50% reduction in mean vitreous haze as compared to 29% in placebo recipients. At the primary endpoint of 26 weeks, 64% of the subjects in the 0.4 mg/kg b.i.d. group demonstrated an improvement of at least 2 grades in vitreous haze or a grade of ≤1+ in the study eye. In the placebo group, this rate was not higher than 46% [48].

In the LX211-02 (Treatment of Clinically Controlled Intermediate and Posterior Uveitis, and Panuveitis) study, the treatment with voclosporin 0.4 mg/kg b.i.d. resulted in a 50% reduction in the rate of inflammatory exacerbations at the 26-week primary end point compared to treatment with placebo. Analysis of the 50-week data from the study's extension period has also provided a similar result. Nearly 90% of subjects were receiving one or more forms of systemic IMT prior to randomization. All patients using IMT have the drug discontinued prior to the beginning of the study. The oral corticotherapy as monotherapy represented nearly 35% of subjects previously using IMT. Additional 30% of subjects were receiving both oral corticosteroids and another immunomodulatory agent, and 28% were being treated with IMT alone [47, 48].

In the LX211-03 (Treatment of Active Anterior Uveitis) study, all treatment groups, including placebo, experienced an improvement in anterior chamber inflammation, resulting in no discernible treatment effect [47, 48].

Potential Risks and Benefits of Voclosporin

Dosage appears to be an important factor in the safety profile of voclosporin. The LX211 studies have demonstrated that 0.4 mg/kg b.i.d. dose is representative of expected risk and is recommended for use in patients with uveitis if voclosporin is approved by the FDA. Relative to placebo, therapy with voclosporin at 0.4 mg/kg b.i.d. roughly halves a patient's exposure to ocular inflammatory insults that lead to loss of vision and to potentially damaging exposure to high rescue doses of corticosteroids. Also, the LX211 studies have shown that treatment with voclosporin permits concomitant withdrawal of other IMTs, allows the reduction of systemic corticosteroid therapy to 5 mg/day or less of prednisone (or its equivalent), and elimination of topical corticosteroid therapy. Moreover, the need for high-dose corticosteroid rescue therapy is avoided and preservation of vision is achieved. Additional benefits may also result from improved control of inflammation, as seen in the voclosporin treatment arms relative to the placebo control, accrued with use of voclosporin in noninfectious uveitis [48].

The percentage of subjects with cataract formation in the study eye, or worsening as per Age-Related Eye Disease Study Lens Grading protocol, was less significant in the two highest voclosporin dose groups than in the placebo group at all assessment times and in all three studies. This finding might reflect a decrease in the usage of corticosteroids and/or a decrease in ocular inflammation [48].

The most common adverse events reported with voclosporin with frequency rates of >5% and at least 2% higher than placebo, regardless of causality, were hypertension, diarrhea, decreased renal function, pyrexia and arthralgia. The time of onset of decreased renal function and hypertension was less than 4 months. When encountered, decreased renal function was reversible with discontinuation of therapy, and hypertensive changes were generally mild to moderate in nature. The effect of moderate CYP 3A4/5 inhibitors on the pharmacokinetics of voclosporin has not been studied; however, an increase in exposure to voclosporin would be expected in the presence of these agents. Caution is recommended when voclosporin is coadministered with moderate CYP 3A4/5 inhibitors and alternative agents should be considered [48].

Voclosporin is currently being evaluated in a second phase 3 study for active non-infectious intermediate, posterior, and pan-uveitis in order to obtain registration for its use and application in uveitis.

m-TOR Pathway Modulator: Sirolimus

Sirolimus, also known as rapamycin, is a natural antibiotic isolated in the 1970s from *Streptomyces hygroscopicus* in the soil samples from Easter Island [11]. It is a cyclic macrolide, a potent immunosuppressant, and an antiangiogenic agent clinically approved for the prevention of solid organ transplant rejection [12, 49]. Similar to tacrolimus and cyclosporine, it is an inhibitor of T cell activation. However, the action of sirolimus differs from that of CsA, blocking either Ca^{2+}-dependent and Ca^{2+}-independent pathways. As a result, it can be used in conjunction with cyclosporin with an additive effect in preventing organ rejection [50].

Rapamycin bioactivity results from the binding to the FK binding protein-12. The resulting complex inhibits the actions of a multifunctional serine-threonine kinase, the mammalian target of rapamycin (mTOR), by specifically binding to its mTORC1 complex [51]. The mTORC1 complex orchestrates multiple basic cellular functions such as cell growth, cell proliferation, cell survival, cell mobility, nutrient levels, reaction to oxidative stress and angiogenesis [52, 53]. The inhibition of mTOR results in G1 cell cycle arrest blocking the cell cycle from G1 to S phase in various cell types, including T and B lymphocytes [49]. It blocks not only cell proliferation but also the expression of signal molecules such as proliferative factors, inflammatory cytokines and ILs like IL-2, IL-4, and IL-15 [54]. By a separate mechanism, in the presence of activated mTOR, the regulatory-associated protein of mTOR (Raptor) activates the hypoxia-inducible factor 1α (HIF-1α), a transcription factor that regulates the VEGF transcription [55]. Rapamycin was shown to increase the rate of HIF-1α degradation in hypoxic environment, to decrease the VEGF production and to reduce vessel response to VEGF15 [56, 57]. The drug also influences the pathway of other pro-angiogenic factors as β-fibroblast growth factor, platelet-derived growth factor-β, nitric oxide synthase, and angiopoietin [56].

The inhibitors of mTOR are expected to show a therapeutic effect in several eye conditions. Dry eye, noninfectious uveitis, and choroidal neovascularization (CNV) are some examples of diseases that may benefit from sirolimus therapy. Several rapamycin-related compounds are in phase I, II and III clinical trials for oncologic patients and for patients suffering of eye conditions. Sirolimus is the active pharmaceutical ingredient in 2 products approved by the FDA, specifically Rapamune®, an immunosuppressive agent used in renal transplant patients, and the CYPHER® sirolimus-eluting coronary stent approved for improving coronary luminal diameter in patients with symptomatic ischemic disease due to its effect on smooth cell and arteries intimal thickening [58–61]. MacuSight Inc. previously had developed the proprietary formulations MS-R001 and MS-R002 for the treatment of ocular diseases. The formulations provide drug exposure to the retina and choroid for up of 2 months, and are amenable to delivery by both ITV and subconjunctival (SCJ) routes of administration [62]. The rights to proprietary formulations MS-R001 and MS-R002 for the treatment of ocular diseases have been transferred from MacuSight to Santen Pharmaceuticals.

Evaluation of Sirolimus Efficacy

Shanmuganathan et al. [62] have used systemic sirolimus as an alternative to treat severe noninfectious uveitis refractory to other drugs or requiring high doses of corticosteroids (systemically or locally). Sirolimus was effective as a corticosteroid-sparing drug in 5 of 8 patients, although in 3 patients the side effects were intolerable or the drug failed to control the uveitis.

A pilot trial conducted by Sen et al. [63] to evaluate the safety and efficacy of subconjunctival sirolimus in 5 patients with active and recalcitrant anterior uveitis has shown no side effects. In this study, 3 patients have shown a two-step decrease in the inflammation and one patient a one-step decrease in the inflammatory process within 4 weeks. Evidence of recurrence was not seen within the following 4 months.

A phase I randomized open-label trial, the SAVE study (Sirolimus as a Therapeutic Approach for Noninfectious Uveitis), is being conducted in the US to evaluate the safety, tolerability and bioactivity of sirolimus given by two different routes of administration, ITV and SCJ [64]. The SAVE study enrolled 30 patients with noninfectious uveitis anatomically classified as posterior, intermediate, and panuveitis. The trial stratified the patients into 3 categories: (1) active uveitis and receiving no treatment; (2) active and receiving corticosteroids equivalent to prednisone >10 mg/day and/or at least 1 other systemic immunosuppressant, and (3) inactive uveitis receiving corticosteroids equivalent to prednisone <10 mg/day and/or at least 1 other systemic immunosuppressant. Patients in each category were randomized into one of two treatment arms, differing in dose and route of administration: (1) ITV injection of 352 μg sirolimus or (2) SCJ injection of 1,320 μg sirolimus. At the primary end point of the SAVE study (6 months), both

SCJ and ITV sirolimus were able to induce complete or partial control of the uveitic activity, as well as to reduce or prevent recurrences of disease. Local administrations of sirolimus, SCJ or ITV, were shown to be safe in patients with noninfectious uveitis. No drug-associated ocular or systemic adverse events were noted. Thus, sirolimus, delivered ocularly, either SCJ or ITV, appears to possess bioactivity as an IMT and steroid-sparing agent in reducing vitreous haze and cells, improving VA, and in decreasing the need for systemic CS [65]. Additional phase II and III studies to evaluate the role of ITV sirolimus in the management of uveitis are currently being conducted.

Potential Risks and Side Effects of Sirolimus

Significant adverse events associated with systemic use of sirolimus have been reported. Hepatobiliary disorders, epidermal and dermal pathologies such as squamous cells carcinoma and photosensitivity, infections, renal, and respiratory disorders are among the most related adverse events reported to the FDA [61]. However, thus far, no drug-related adverse events have been established with intraocular or SCJ application of this drug [65].

Biologics

Among the most recent therapies for uveitis are the biologics, also known as biologic response modifiers [28]. The targets of these drugs are specific cytokines or their receptors involved in the inflammatory pathways. Several of these drugs are antibodies that target directly the cytokines such as TNF, or the IL receptors such as IL-2 receptor, and or a ligand such as the B cell surface antigen CD-2019 [39]. They are typically used in the treatment of malignancy, inducing stimulation of the immune system [66]. The results in the treatment of noninfectious uveitis have generally been positive in patients with history of poor visual outcomes despite immunosuppressive therapy [39]. Tumor necrosis factor-α inhibitors (infliximab, etanercept, and adalimumab), antilymphocyte agents (rituximab and alemtuzumab), and an IL-2 receptor blocker (daclizumab) are the biologic response modifiers that have been used to treat uveitis [40]. Recombinant IL-10 has been shown to attenuate inflammatory conditions as well as downregulate ocular inflammation or to contribute to a higher threshold of resistance to uveitis. IL-1 trap has also demonstrated therapeutic efficacy in inflammatory conditions.

Inhibitors of IL-1: Rilonacept, Canakinumab, Anakinra, and Gevokizumab

It is becoming increasingly apparent that innate immunity plays a determinant role in previously considered autoimmune diseases. Pattern recognition receptors, namely toll-like receptors (TLRs) and nucleotide oligomerization domain (NOD)-like receptors (NLRs), are central to the induction of innate immunity through their capacity to detect pathogen-associated molecular patterns (PAMPs) [67]. PAMPs that trigger innate responses have also been implicated in the induction of autoinflammatory responses in several diseases associated with uveitis, such as sarcoidosis [68], Behçet's disease [69], reactive arthritis [70], ankylosing spondylitis [71], and inflammatory bowel disease. TLRs are expressed within the eye [67]. Controlling uveitis with TLR4 agonist lipopolysaccharide has been discussed [72, 73]. NLRs are just as likely as TLRs to be crucial participants in the basic immunologic mechanisms involved in uveitis. Indeed, NLR family members have been identified as the genetic link between diverse autoinflammatory diseases [74, 75]. NOD1 plays an important role in host defense and recognizes the minimal component of bacterial cell walls, meso-diaminopimelic acid. Polymorphisms in *NOD1* are associated with autoinflammatory diseases characterized by uveitis such as Crohn's disease and sarcoidosis. NOD1 is homologous to NOD2, which is responsible for an autosomal dominant form of uveitis. NOD1, NOD2 and NOD-like receptor called NLR, are expressed within uveitic eyes, resulting in uncontrolled inflammation in an IL-1β-dependent mechanism [76]. NOD-1 induces the production of IL-1 in the eye in a caspase-1-dependent mechanism. Deficiency in caspase-1 or IL-1 type I receptor (IL-1RI) abrogated uveitis, identifying the IL-1-signaling pathway as an essential downstream mediator of NOD1-triggered ocular inflammation. This is in contrast to NOD2, which promotes IL-1 synthesis through caspase-1 but does not require IL-1 signaling events for the development of uveitis [77]. The NLRP-3 gene encodes the protein cryopyrin, an important component of the inflammatory cascade. Cryopyrin regulates the protease caspase-1 and controls the activation of IL-1β. Mutations in NLRP-3 result in an overactive inflammasome resulting in excessive release of activated IL-1β that drives inflammation.

IL-1 is a proinflammatory cytokine known to play a crucial role in chronic inflammation. This IL is involved in T helper cell costimulation, B cell maturation and proliferation, NK cell activation and a small amount induces acute phase reaction [78]. IL-1β is one of the major cytokines implicated in the pathogenesis of many inflammatory-associated diseases [78]. IL-1β was also shown to play an important role in uveitis associated with juvenile idiopathic arthritis and Behcet's disease (BD). IL-1β is, therefore, becoming a focus for the development of new anti-inflammatory drug products. Currently, there are four types of IL-1β blockade compounds, namely anti-IL-1β antibody, IL-1 receptor antagonists such as sIL-1Ra and icIL-1Ra and IL1 trap [78]. Canakinumab (Ilaris®, Novartis) and Anakinra (Kineret®) have been approved by FDA to treat rheumatic disease and have brought benefits to patients [78]. Anakinra is also approved to treat pain and swelling in rheumatoid arthritis [79]. Rilonacept (ARCALYST®, Regeneron) has been approved for the management of cryopyrin-associated periodic syndromes (CAPS), a group of rare diseases that include familial cold autoinflammatory syndrome and Muckle-Wells syndrome, secondary to mutations on the gene that codify the NLRP-3.

Rilonacept (ARCALYST)

Rilonacept is a recombinant fusion protein consisting of human cytokine receptor extracellular domains and the Fc portion of human IgG1 designed to block the signaling pathway of IL-1 [80]. Rilonacept incorporates in a single molecule the extracellular domains of both receptor components required for IL-1 signaling: the IL-1RI and the IL-1 receptor accessory protein. Since it contains both receptor components, rilonacept binds IL-1 with picomolar affinity. Despite binding the endogenous receptor antagonist, rilonacept readily blocks IL-1-induced gene expression and histopathological changes in vivo [80].

Bioactivity. The injection of human IL-1 into C57BL/6 mice caused a rapid rise in serum IL-6 levels that peaked at 2 h. Administration of human rilonacept 24 h before IL-1 completely blocked the subsequent induction of IL-6 [80]. Studies were conducted in healthy volunteers and in patients with autoimmune diseases. In the efficacy study with 23 patients, which evaluated the long-term efficacy and safety of once-weekly dosing (160 mg) of rilonacept in patients with CAPS, rilonacept markedly and rapidly decreased the clinical signs and symptoms of CAPS (rash, feeling of fever/chills, joint pain, eye redness/pain, and fatigue) [79]. Therefore, ARCALYST (rilonacept) injection for SC was approved in February 2008 in the United States for the treatment of CAPS, including Familial Cold Auto-inflammatory Syndrome and Muckle-Wells Syndrome in adults and children age 12 and older.

Potential Risks and Side Effects. Rilonacept was generally well tolerated. Across all studies, injection site reactions were the most common adverse events associated with subcutaneous use of rilonacept. Treatment-emergent infections such as atypical mycobacterial infection, gastrointestinal hemorrhage and colitis, sinusitis, and bronchitis, were the next most commonly reported type of adverse events [80].

Application in Uveitis and Ocular Inflammatory Diseases. Rilonacept is being investigated in a proof-of-concept clinical trial for noninfectious intermediate, posterior, and pan-uveitis.

Canakinumab (Ilaris)

Canakinumab is a human monoclonal IgG1/κ isotype antibody that binds to the human IL-1β and neutralizes its activity by blocking its interaction with IL-1 receptors, but it does not bind IL-1α or IL-1α receptor antagonist (IL-1RA) [81]. ILARIS may be associated with an increased risk of serious infections, predominantly of upper respiratory tract. Other side effects are nasopharyngitis, diarrhea, influenza, headache and nausea [81].

Application in Uveitis and Ocular Inflammatory Diseases. Although it may be a very good candidate, canakinumab has not been evaluated in clinical trials for uveitis. Perhaps it can be considered in the future so that canakinumab may have the opportunity to play a role in the management of ocular inflammatory diseases.

Anakinra (Kineret)

Anakinra is a recombinant nonglycosylated form of the human IL-1RA. It blocks the biologic activity of IL-1 by competitively inhibiting IL-1 binding to the IL-1RI. The safety and efficacy of Kineret have been evaluated in three randomized, double-masked, placebo-controlled trials of 1,392 patients ≥18 years of age with active rheumatoid arthritis [82]. The most common and consistently reported treatment-related adverse event associated with Kineret is injection site reaction like redness, swelling, bruising, itching, pain and stinging. An increased rate of infections was also reported [82].

Application in Uveitis and Ocular Inflammatory Diseases. Anakinra has not been evaluated in clinical trials for noninfectious intermediate, posterior, and pan-uveitis. However, it has been used by uveitis specialists in selected cases of refractory posterior uveitis as well as cases of juvenile idiopathic arthritis-associated uveitis.

Gevokizumab

XOMA and Servier have agreed to jointly develop and commercialize the IL-1β-targeted monoclonal antibody gevokizumab (XOMA 052) for the treatment of multiple inflammatory disorders and vascular diseases [83]. In 2010, XOMA/Servier announced positive results from an open-label pilot study of XOMA 052 in BD patients with refractive uveitis. In this study, all 7 patients enrolled in the trial displayed reduction in intraocular inflammation and improvement in visual acuity. Five patients received a second infusion to blunt a developing exacerbation, and all responded to the second infusion. The drug appeared to be safe for ocular use, and no drug-related adverse events were reported [84]. Gevokizumab is currently undergoing phase II trials in diabetes type II and cardiovascular disease.

Application in Uveitis and Ocular Inflammatory Diseases. Gevokizumab has not been formally evaluated in clinical trials for noninfectious intermediate, posterior, and pan-uveitis, except for the uveitis associated with BD. Hopefully, the pilot data will be sufficiently supportive for future trials in uveitis.

Inhibitor of IL-6: Tocilizumab

IL-6 is a pleiotropic inflammatory cytokine produced by T cells, monocytes, and macrophages. IL-6, also referred to as B cell stimulatory factor-2 and interferon-β_2, is a cytokine involved in a wide variety of biological functions. It plays an essential role in the final differentiation of B cells into Ig-secreting cells, as well as inducing myeloma/plasmacytoma growth, nerve cell differentiation, and, in hepatocytes, acute-phase reactants, such as hepcidin and C-reactive protein. It is essential for the differentiation of Th17 subset involved in uveitis. High levels of IL-6 in the vitreous of patients with refractory/chronic uveitis have been reported by Yoshimura et al. [85]. They have shown that systemic administration of an IL-6 antibody ameliorates EAU by suppressing both the systemic and regional Th17 response. Haruta et al. [86] and Hohki et al. [87] have also demonstrated in animal studies that inhibition of IL-6 leads to suppression of EAU via inhibition of Th17 cells.

Tocilizumab, commercialized under the name of ACTEMRA/RoACTEMRA, is a humanized IgG1 monoclonal antibody against both soluble and membrane-bound IL-6 receptors (sIL-6R and mIL-6R) [88]. Tocilizumab was approved by the FDA in 2010 to treat rheumatoid arthritis in patients who have been refractory to other therapies. Clinical studies in RA patients have shown benefits in reducing joint inflammation, joint damage, and fatigue [89, 90]. This drug has also been effective in the treatment of patients with severe systemic-onset form of juvenile idiopathic arthritis and vasculitis syndromes [91–93]. It is the first monoclonal antibody which targets IL-6 and offers an alternative to 30% of arthritis patients not responding to or intolerant of TNF blockers [90, 94]. The efficacy of ACTEMRA/RoACTEMRA in alleviating the signs and symptoms of RA was assessed in five randomized, double-masked, multicenter phase III studies: the AMBITON Study, the LITHE Study, the OPTION Study, the TOWARD Study, and the RADIATE Study [88–90, 94, 95]. In total, the studies enrolled more than 4,200 patients with moderate to severe RA around the world, with the results being consistent with the effect of IL-6 on acute-phase reactants. Treatment with tocilizumab was associated with rapid decreases in C-reactive protein and increases in hemoglobin levels. A joint effort by Roche, Chugai, and Genentech has developed and commercialized the drug. The adverse drug reactions of tocilizumab are presented in table 2 and are based on the safety reported in the five studies of ACTEMRA/RoACTEMRA.

Application in Uveitis and Ocular Inflammatory Diseases. Tocilizumab is being investigated in a proof-of-concept clinical trial for noninfectious intermediate, posterior, and pan-uveitis.

The Immune System as a Potential Target of New Drugs

Currently, several compounds targeting different molecules in the inflammatory cascades are being tested for rheumatic diseases. These agents may represent potential therapeutic options, through proper clinical trials, for ocular diseases such as uveitis and are listed in table 3.

Novel Drug Delivery Systems

Given the potential side effects associated with systemic therapies, the unmet needs in the field of uveitis and ocular inflammatory diseases are new drug delivery systems that can aid in decreasing systemic side effects, allowing rapid local delivery of high concentration of drug, and ensuring a sustained local release of the pharmacologic agents. Among the new approaches are the applications of nanoparticles and iontophoresis.

Nanoparticles

A particle ranging in size from 1 to 1,000 nm that behaves as a whole unit in terms of its physical properties is called an ultrafine or nanoparticle. From a cream that

Table 2. Systemic adverse events of ACTEMRA

Infections and infestations	Upper respiratory tract infections, cellulitis, pneumonia, oral herpes simplex, herpes zoster, diverticulitis
Gastrointestinal disorders	Abdominal pain, mouth ulceration, gastritis, stomatitis, gastric ulcer
Skin and subcutaneous tissue disorders	Rash, pruritus, urticaria
Nervous system disorders	Headache, dizziness
Investigations	Hepatic transaminases increased, weight increased, total bilirubin increased
Vascular disorders	Hypertension
Blood and lymphatic system disorders	Leukopenia, neutropenia
Metabolism and nutrition disorders	Hypercholesterolemia, hypertriglyceridemia
General disorders and administration site conditions	Peripheral edema hypersensitivity reactions
Eye disorders	Conjunctivitis
Renal disorders	Nephrolithiasis
Endocrine disorders	Hypothyroidism

releases nitric oxide gas to combat *Staphylococcus* infection to quantum dots that identify location of cancer cells in the body, the potential uses of nanoparticles are countless. And rightly so, nanoparticles have been a focal point of research focusing on development of better drug delivery mechanisms.

Nanoparticles are classified into nanospheres and nanocapsules depending on the spatial arrangement of the drug to the particles matrix (fig. 3). Nanospheres are solid spheres consisting of dense solid polymeric network, developing over a large specific area. Drugs can be either incorporated into the matrix of the nanospheres or adsorbed onto the surface of the colloidal carrier. Nanocapsules, on the other hand, are small containers formed of a central cavity surrounded by a polymeric membrane [96].

The use of nanoparticles has been investigated in managing conditions such as glaucoma and infectious and noninfectious uveitis [97–101]. In order to treat an anterior segment condition, the drug-loaded nanoparticles are instilled topically in the cul-de-sac of the eye, from where the drug is slowly released into the lacrimal pool by disintegration of the polymer matrix. The success of a nanoparticle drug delivery system for ophthalmic use depends upon the physical and structural properties of the polymer, which in turn dictates its rate of degradation. Currently, there is a lack

Table 3. Therapeutic agents to be considered for uveitis and ocular inflammatory diseases

Cytokines	
New TNF-α blockers	
Certolizumab pegol (Cimizia®)	The drug is a PEGylated molecule of the Fab portion of a monoclonal immunoglobulin against TNF-α. It was approved by FDA to treat Crohn's disease and rheumatoid arthritis.
Golimumab (Simponi®)	The human monoclonal antibody against TNF-α was designed for monthly injections. It was approved by FDA to treat rheumatoid arthritis, psoriatic arthritis, and ankylosing spondylitis.
ESBA105CRD04	An exploratory study with this new TNF blocker for topical use in anterior uveitis is being conducted in Germany.
Interleukin	
IL-15	
AMG714 (HuMax-IL15)	The index human monoclonal IgG1 against the IL-15 neutralizes both exogenous and endogenous IL-15 activity in vitro. IL-15 acts similarly to IL-2 and induces proliferation of natural killer cells.
IL-17	
AIN457	The human monoclonal IgG1 targets IL-17 with high affinity, neutralizing the bioactivity of this cytokine.
Ligands	
VCAM-1/VLA-4	
Natalizumab	The humanized monoclonal IgG4-antibody targets the α_4-integrin subunit of VLA-4. It blocks the binding of VLA-4 to VCAM-1 and interferes with an important molecular interaction for the entry of leukocytes into sites of inflammation.
ICAM-1	
ISIS-2302	The 20-nucleotide phosphorothioate antisense oligonucleotide was designed to inhibit the expression of ICAM-1. It can block the ICAM-1 transcription, which reduces its expression levels and thus prevents the entry of leukocytes into sites of inflammation.
ICAM-1/ LFA-1	
Efalizumab	Another inhibitor of the ICAM-1/LFA-1 axis is the index humanized monoclonal IgG1 antibody. It binds the CD11, a chain of LFA-1, and therefore blocks interaction with ICAM-1.
Receptors	
CTLA4-Ig	
Abatacept (belatacept)	The fusion protein blocks the receptor on APCs and thus prevents costimulation of T cells, resulting in immunosuppression by blocking T cell activation.
CD-20	

Table 3. Continued

Rituximab	The monoclonal chimeric antibody acts against the CD20 expressed on B cells. Anti-CD20 therapy affects the secretion of proinflammatory cytokines, antigen presentation, T cell activation, and autoantibody production.
CD-52	
Alemtuzumab (Campath-1H)	The humanized monoclonal antibody targets the CD-52. Even a single treatment can substantially deplete the blood of lymphocytes, resulting in leukopenia that can last for several months.
Complement cascade (innate immune system)	
POT-4	The compound is a cyclic peptide that binds and inactivates complement component 3, which is essential for the formation of the membrane attack complex. The drug has been tested in a dose escalating phase I study for subfoveal CNV, and has the potential to be used in uveitis once the safety and tolerability results encourage its use.
ARC1905	The compound is a PEGylated RNA aptamer that inhibits the complement component 5, blocking the formation of the membrane attack complex.

of data regarding the use of nanoparticle administration to treat a posterior segment condition. Data from animal studies by Bourges et al. [102] have shown a sustained release of the drug (tamoxifen) from nanoparticles 4 months after a single injection of nanoparticles for the treatment of experimental autoimmune uveoretinitis (EAU). The authors showed that rats injected with tamoxifen-loaded nanoparticles did not develop EAU compared to the group injected with free drug.

There is currently no nanoparticle formulation in clinical trials for uveitis and other diseases; however, animal studies have shown promising results [103]. Microspheres of PKC412 (protein C inhibitor) and inhibitors of receptors for VEGF have been successfully used in treating CNV [104]. Other investigators have shown successful reduction in development of experimental proliferative vitreoretinopathy using 5-FU and Ara-C combination nanoparticles [105–107].

The goal of therapy for uveitis is to eliminate inflammation in the eye, reduce frequency of recurrences, decrease or avoid systemic and ocular adverse events associated with therapy, and improve quality of life. Nanoparticles may have the potential to deliver on all these important goals.

Iontophoresis for Uveitis

With unique physicochemical properties, each drug will have varying abilities to penetrate ocular tissue, diffuse into the posterior chamber, and remain at therapeutic

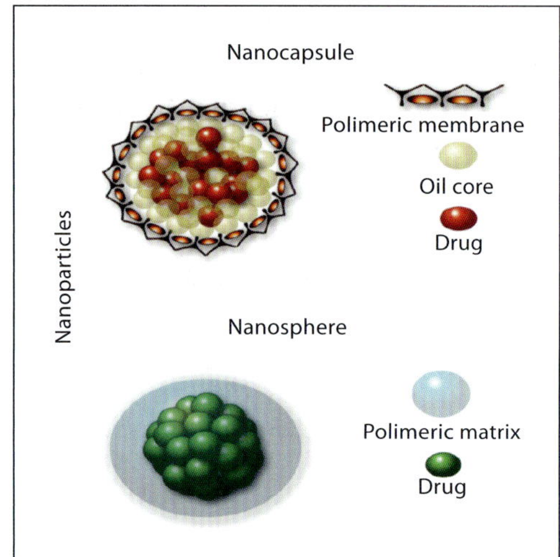

Fig. 3. Schematic representation of the spatial relationship between drug and nanoparticles in nanospheres and nanocapsules.

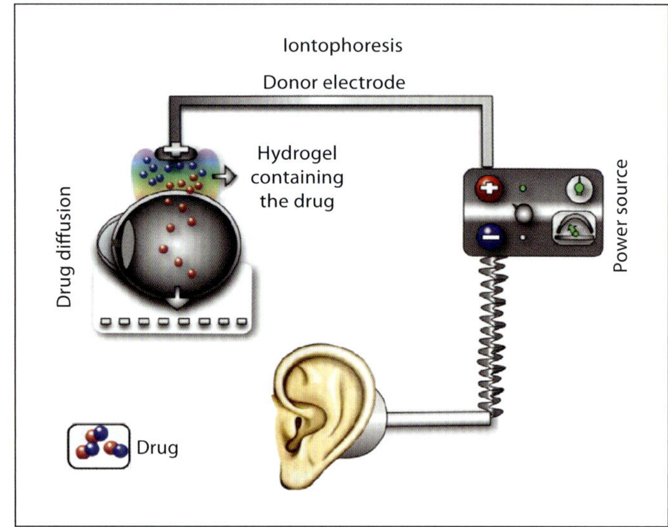

Fig. 4. Schematic representation of a simple iontophoresis device applied to deliver a positively charged drug. The donor electrode containing the drug carrying the same charge as the electrode is placed on the eye, and the return electrode is placed on another body surface. The drug serves as a conductor of the current through the ocular tissues.

doses before being eliminated. Iontophoresis is a noninvasive technique used to enhance the penetration of ionic drug through tissue using a low electric current (fig. 4). This mode of drug delivery provides a potential alternative to minimize the complications related to intraocular injections and increase the bioavailability of topically administered drugs. Ocular iontophoresis was studied extensively in the first half of the 20th century. However, the lack of randomized controlled trials and the paucity of toxicity data led to it being sidelined as a drug delivery mechanism. As the beginning of the 21st century saw an increased interest in development of newer efficient modes of drug delivery, iontophoresis once again came into the lime light for safe and quick delivery of high concentration of drugs to specific sites. Iontophoresis has been most widely used to deliver transdermal local anesthetics and antibiotics. In 1908, a German scientist Wirtz used iontophoresis to treat corneal ulcers, keratitis and episcleritis, and his initial work inspired others to investigate the pharmacokinetics, penetration and efficacy of numerous antibiotics. However, the advent of newer potent topical preparation of these antimicrobials led to the demise of this approach.

Iontophoresis enhances drug delivery via electrophoresis (enhanced movement of ionic species by the applied electric field), electro-osmosis (transport of both neutral and charged species by an electric field-induced convective solvent flow) and electroporation (alteration of the tissue barrier that increases the intrinsic permeability of the membrane) [108–111]. Based on the site of treatment, iontophoresis is classified into transcorneal and transscleral. Transcorneal iontophoresis has mainly been used to deliver drugs to the anterior segment across the corneal layers while transscleral iontophoresis overcomes lens-iris barrier and delivers drugs directly into the vitreous and retina through the choroid or indirectly through systemic circulation or anterior chamber.

Evaluations in animal models of drugs delivered via transscleral iontophoresis reveal differential pharmacokinetic profiles, particularly when ITV drug concentration and duration are the measured parameters [103]. For example, using a current of 2.0 mA/0.5 cm^2 and duration of 10 min, methyl-prednisolone reached a peak concentration of 45 μg/ml 2 h after application, maintaining greater tissue concentration than the same dose delivered intravenously [112]. In anti-infectious control, the antibiotic gentamicin saw a peak concentration of 53.5 μg/ml in the vitreous at 16 h following transscleral iontophoresis, still significantly higher than levels achieved with SCJ injection [108]. Administration for 10 min at 1 mA of foscarnet, used to treat cytomegalovirus infection, resulted in a peak concentration after only 4 h, but maintenance of therapeutic levels for up to 60 h following iontophoresis, indicating a slower elimination rate than other drugs delivered via the same method [113]. These results suggest that different drugs behave differently in the same electromagnetic environment. Early-phase studies employing iontophoresis as the method of drug delivery in patients with various forms of ocular inflammation have shown encouraging results. In a phase II clinical trial, Chauvaud et al. [114] has shown that methylprednisolone hemiscuccinate (SoluMedrol) was well tolerated, safe, and reduced the need of systemic corticosteroids. Patients with acute corneal graft rejection have also received corticosteroids once daily for 3 consecutive days (1.5 mA 3 min) via the same mechanism in addition to topical steroids and have shown improvement in visual acuity and elimination of need for analgesics [115, 116].

Although iontophoresis is a relatively safe technique of drug delivery, one should be aware that at high current densities of 100–700 mA/cm^2, adverse reactions such as retinal and choroidal burns, hemorrhagic necrosis, edema, and infiltrations have been observed. Tissue damage can also occur with an increased duration of the procedure. The extent of such damage depends on the site of the application and current density.

Application in Uveitis and Ocular Inflammatory Diseases
Iontophoresis technology has been evaluated for uveitis. The early study using dexamethasone as the index drug delivered via iontophoresis has demonstrated safety and bioactivity in patients' anterior uveitis. Such success has led to the multicenter phase 3 study evaluating dexamethasone phosphate delivered by ocular iontophoresis [4.0 mA-min at 1.5 mA compared to iontophoresis with sodium citrate buffer solution (100 mM) 4.0 mA-min at similar current] for noninfectious anterior uveitis currently being conducted in the United States.

Conclusions

Patients with uveitis and ocular inflammatory diseases are in desperate need of effective therapeutic agents which not only eliminate inflammation and prevent recurrences but also protect the patients from potential side effects. In addition, we believe that all currently available drugs should be approved by the regulatory bodies as soon as possible so that they can be of benefit to all patients.

The horizon currently appears very bright, given the many therapeutic agents and approaches for uveitis and ocular inflammatory diseases. Different classes of agents, from calcineurin inhibitors to mTOR inhibitors and IL inhibitors, among others, are being evaluated. In addition, delivery systems such as iontophoresis will also allow novel methods of safe and effective administration of pharmacologic agents. Hopefully, such efforts will lead to therapeutic options for our patients in the near future.

References

1 Jabs DA, Nussenblatt RB, Rosenbaum JT: Standardization of uveitis nomenclature for reporting clinical data. Results of the First International Workshop. Am J Ophthalmol 2005;140:509–516.
2 Whitcup S: Uveitis 2003: Diagnosis and Management of Ocular Inflammation in the 21st Century: The uveitic syndromes – autoimmune and posterior uveitis: sarcoidosis. Uveitis Subspecialty Day Program and abstracts of the American Academy of Ophthalmology 2003 Annual Meeting, Anaheim, November 2003.
3 Loh AR, Acharya NR: Incidence rates and risk factors for ocular complications and vision loss in HLA-B27-associated uveitis. Am J Ophthalmol 2010; 150:534e2–542e2.
4 Gritz DC, Wong IG: Incidence and prevalence of uveitis in Northern California; the Northern California Epidemiology of Uveitis Study. Ophthalmology 2004;17:491–500.
5 Nussenblatt RB: The natural history of uveitis. Int Ophthalmol 1990;14:303–308.
6 Darrell RW, Wagener HP, Kurland LT: Epidemiology of uveitis. Incidence and prevalence in a small urban community. Arch Ophthalmol 1962;68:502–514.
7 Suttorp-Schulten MS, Rothova A: The possible impact of uveitis in blindness: a literature survey. Br J Ophthalmol 1996;80:844–848.
8 Suhler EB, Lloyd MJ, Choi D, Rosenbaum JT, Austin DF: Incidence and prevalence of uveitis in Veterans Affairs Medical Centers of the Pacific Northwest. Am J Ophthalmol 2008;146:890e8–896e8.
9 Durrani OM, Tehrani NN, Marr JE, Moradi P, Stavrou P, Murray PI: Degree, duration, and causes of visual loss in uveitis. Br J Ophthalmol 2004;88: 1159–1162.

10 Beraud E, Kotake S, Caspi RR, et al: Control of experimental autoimmune uveoretinitis by low dose T cell vaccination. Cell Immunol 1992;140:112–122.
11 Pennesi G, Caspi RR: Genetic control of susceptibility in clinical and experimental uveitis. Int Rev Immunol 2002;21:67–88.
12 Heiligenhaus A, Thurau S, Hennig M, Grajewski RS, Wildner G: Anti-inflammatory treatment of uveitis with biologicals: new treatment options that reflect pathogenetic knowledge of the disease. Graefes Arch Clin Exp Ophthalmol 2010;248:1531–1551.
13 Hoekzema R, Murray PI, van Haren MA, Helle M, Kijlstra A: Analysis of interleukin-6 in endotoxin-induced uveitis. Invest Ophthalmol Vis Sci 1991; 32:88–95.
14 Ohta K, Yamagami S, Taylor AW, Streilein JW: IL-6 antagonizes TGF-beta and abolishes immune privilege in eyes with endotoxin-induced uveitis. Invest Ophthalmol Vis Sci 2000;41:2591–2599.
15 Caspi R: Autoimmunity in the immune privileged eye: pathogenic and regulatory T cells. Immunol Res 2008;42:41–50.
16 von Toerne C, Sieg C, Kaufmann U, Diedrichs-Mohring M, Nelson PJ, Wildner G: Effector T cells driving monophasic vs. relapsing/remitting experimental autoimmune uveitis show unique pathway signatures. Mol Immunol 2010;48:272–280.
17 Horai R, Caspi RR: Cytokines in autoimmune uveitis. J Interferon Cytokine Res 2011;31:733–744.
18 Barton K, McLauchlan MT, Calder VL, Lightman S: The kinetics of cytokine mRNA expression in the retina during experimental autoimmune uveoretinitis. Cell Immunol 1995;164:133–140.
19 Haruta H, Ohguro N, Fujimoto M, et al: Blockade of interleukin-6 signaling suppresses not only th17 but also interphotoreceptor retinoid binding protein-specific Th1 by promoting regulatory T cells in experimental autoimmune uveoretinitis. Invest Ophthalmol Vis Sci 2011;52:3264–3271.
20 Ishida W, Fukuda K, Higuchi T, Kajisako M, Sakamoto S, Fukushima A: Dynamic changes of microRNAs in the eye during the development of experimental autoimmune uveoretinitis. Invest Ophthalmol Vis Sci 2011;52:611–617.
21 Jha P, Sohn JH, Xu Q, et al: The complement system plays a critical role in the development of experimental autoimmune anterior uveitis. Invest Ophthalmol Vis Sci 2006;47:1030–1038.
22 Charteris DG, Barton K, McCartney AC, Lightman SL: CD4+ lymphocyte involvement in ocular Behcet's disease. Autoimmunity 1992;12:201–206.
23 George RK, Chan CC, Whitcup SM, Nussenblatt RB: Ocular immunopathology of Behcet's disease. Surv Ophthalmol 1997;42:157–162.
24 Whitcup SM, Chan CC, Li Q, Nussenblatt RB: Expression of cell adhesion molecules in posterior uveitis. Arch Ophthalmol 1992;110:662–666.
25 Durrani OM, Meads CA, Murray PI: Uveitis: a potentially blinding disease. Ophthalmologica 2004; 218:223–236.
26 Pato E, Munoz-Fernandez S, Francisco F, et al: Systematic review on the effectiveness of immunosuppressants and biological therapies in the treatment of autoimmune posterior uveitis. Semin Arthritis Rheum 2011;40:314–323.
27 Jabs DA, Rosenbaum JT, Foster CS, et al: Guidelines for the use of immunosuppressive drugs in patients with ocular inflammatory disorders: recommendations of an expert panel. Am J Ophthalmol 2000; 130:492–513.
28 Larson T, Nussenblatt RB, Sen HN: Emerging drugs for uveitis. Expert Opin Emerg Drugs 2011;16:309–322.
29 Jaffe GJ, Martin D, Callanan D, Pearson PA, Levy B, Comstock T: Fluocinolone acetonide implant (Retisert) for noninfectious posterior uveitis: thirty-four-week results of a multicenter randomized clinical study. Ophthalmology 2006;113:1020–1027.
30 Callanan DG, Jaffe GJ, Martin DF, Pearson PA, Comstock TL: Treatment of posterior uveitis with a fluocinolone acetonide implant: three-year clinical trial results. Arch Ophthalmol 2008;126:1191–1201.
31 Anglade E, Yatscoff R, Foster R, Grau U: Next-generation calcineurin inhibitors for ophthalmic indications. Expert Opin Investig Drugs 2007;16: 1525–1540.
32 Lee RW, Schewitz LP, Nicholson LB, Dayan CM, Dick AD: Steroid refractory CD4+ T cells in patients with sight-threatening uveitis. Invest Ophthalmol Vis Sci 2009;50:4273–4278.
33 Pujari SS, Kempen JH, Newcomb CW, et al: Cyclophosphamide for ocular inflammatory diseases. Ophthalmology 2010;117:356–365.
34 Nguyen QD, Hatef E, Kayen B, et al: A cross-sectional study of the current treatment patterns in noninfectious uveitis among specialists in the United States. Ophthalmology 2011;118:184–190.
35 Ikeda E, Hikita N, Eto K, Mochizuki M: Tacrolimus-rapamycin combination therapy for experimental autoimmune uveoretinitis. Jpn J Ophthalmol 1997; 41:396–402.
36 Kilmartin DJ, Forrester JV, Dick AD: Tacrolimus (FK506) in failed cyclosporin A therapy in endogenous posterior uveitis. Ocul Immunol Inflamm 1998;6:101–109.
37 Sloper CM, Powell RJ, Dua HS: Tacrolimus (FK506) in the treatment of posterior uveitis refractory to cyclosporine. Ophthalmology 1999;106:723–728.

38 Kempen JH, Daniel E, Gangaputra S, et al: Methods for identifying long-term adverse effects of treatment in patients with eye diseases: the Systemic Immunosuppressive Therapy for Eye Diseases (SITE) Cohort Study. Ophthalmic Epidemiol 2008; 15:47–55.
39 Okada AA: The dream of biologics in uveitis. Arch Ophthalmol 2010;128:632–635.
40 Okada AA: Immunomodulatory therapy for ocular inflammatory disease: a basic manual and review of the literature. Ocul Immunol Inflamm 2005;13: 335–351.
41 Dumont F: Cyclosporine A and tacrolimus (FK-506) immunosuppression through immunophilin-dependent inhibition of calcineurin function. In: Lieberman RMA, ed. Principles of Drug Development in Transplantation and Autoimmunity. New York: Chapman and Hall 1996;175–205.
42 Ho S, Clipstone N, Timmermann L, et al: The mechanism of action of cyclosporin A and FK506. Clin Immunol Immunopathol 1996;80:S40–S45.
43 Cho ML, Cho CS, Min SY, et al: Cyclosporine inhibition of vascular endothelial growth factor production in rheumatoid synovial fibroblasts. Arthritis Rheum 2002;46:1202–1209.
44 Schreiber SL, Crabtree GR: The mechanism of action of cyclosporin A and FK506. Immunol Today 1992;13:136–142.
45 Stalder M, Birsan T, Hubble RW, Paniagua RT, Morris RE: In vivo evaluation of the novel calcineurin inhibitor ISATX247 in non-human primates. J Heart Lung Transplant 2003;22:1343–1352.
46 Kuglstatter A, Mueller F, Kusznir E, et al: Structural basis for the cyclophilin A binding affinity and immunosuppressive potency of E-ISA247 (voclosporin). Acta Crystallogr D Biol Crystallogr 2011; 67:119–123.
47 Sepah YJ ME, Metcalf B, Khwaja A, Channa R, Ibrahim M, Hatef E, Heo J, Hee JL, Rentiya ZS DD, Nguyen QD: Voclosporin: a potentially promising therapeutic agent for noninfectious uveitis. Expert Rev Ophthalmol 2011;6:281–286.
48 Anglade E, Aspeslet LJ, Weiss SL: A new agent for the treatment of noninfectious uveitis: rationale and design of three LUMINATE (Lux Uveitis Multicenter Investigation of a New Approach to Treatment) trials of steroid-sparing voclosporin. Clin Ophthalmol 2008;2:693–702.
49 Kahan BD, Podbielski J, Napoli KL, Katz SM, Meier-Kriesche HU, Van Buren CT: Immunosuppressive effects and safety of a sirolimus/cyclosporine combination regimen for renal transplantation. Transplantation 1998;66:1040–1046.
50 Longoria J, Roberts RF, Marboe CC, Stouch BC, Starnes VA, Barr ML: Sirolimus (rapamycin) potentiates cyclosporine in prevention of acute lung rejection. J Thorac Cardiovasc Surg 1999;117:714–718.
51 Sehgal SN: Sirolimus: its discovery, biological properties, and mechanism of action. Transplant Proc 2003;35:7S–14S.
52 Kim DH, Sarbassov DD, Ali SM, et al: mTOR interacts with raptor to form a nutrient-sensitive complex that signals to the cell growth machinery. Cell 2002;110:163–175.
53 Kim DH, Sarbassov DD, Ali SM, et al: GbetaL, a positive regulator of the rapamycin-sensitive pathway required for the nutrient-sensitive interaction between raptor and mTOR. Mol Cell 2003;11:895–904.
54 Sehgal SN: Rapamune (RAPA, rapamycin, sirolimus): mechanism of action immunosuppressive effect results from blockade of signal transduction and inhibition of cell cycle progression. Clin Biochem 1998;31:335–340.
55 Shoshani T, Faerman A, Mett I, et al: Identification of a novel hypoxia-inducible factor 1-responsive gene, RTP801, involved in apoptosis. Mol Cell Biol 2002;22:2283–2293.
56 Attur MG, Patel R, Thakker G, Vyas P, et al: Differential anti-inflammatory effects of immunosuppressive drugs: cyclosporin, rapamycin and FK-506 on inducible nitric oxide synthase, nitric oxide, cyclooxygenase-2 and PGE2 production. Inflamm Res 2000;49:20–26.
57 Kwon YS, Hong HS, Kim JC, Shin JS, Son Y: Inhibitory effect of rapamycin on corneal neovascularization in vitro and in vivo. Invest Ophthalmol Vis Sci 2005;46:454–460.
58 Gregory CR, Huie P, Billingham ME, Morris RE: Rapamycin inhibits arterial intimal thickening caused by both alloimmune and mechanical injury. Its effect on cellular, growth factor, and cytokine response in injured vessels. Transplantation 1993;55: 1409–1418.
59 Guba M, von Breitenbuch P, Steinbauer M, et al: Rapamycin inhibits primary and metastatic tumor growth by antiangiogenesis: involvement of vascular endothelial growth factor. Nat Med 2002;8:128–135.
60 Shuchman M: Trading restenosis for thrombosis? New questions about drug-eluting stents. N Engl J Med 2006;355:1949–1952.
61 Rapamune (package insert). Philadelphia, Wyeth Pharmaceuticals, 2008.
62 Shanmuganathan VA, Casely EM, Raj D, et al: The efficacy of sirolimus in the treatment of patients with refractory uveitis. Br J Ophthalmol 2005;89: 666–669.

63 Nida H, Sen TAL, Meleth AD, Smith WM, Nussenblatt RB: Subconjunctival sirolimus for the treatment of active anterior uveitis: results of a pilot trial, in press.
64 NCT00908466. Cgi. http://clinicaltrialsgov/ct2/show/NCT00908466.
65 Mohamed A, Ibrahim AW, Rentiya Z, Sepah YJ, Leder HA, Hatef E, Naor J, Shams NK, Dunn JP, Nguyen QD: Sirolimus as Therapeutic Approach to Uveitis: A Randomized Study to Assess the Safety and Bioactivity of Intravitreal and Subconjunctival Injections of Sirolimus in Patients with Non-Infectious Uveitis (The Save Study). ARVO, Fort Lauderdale, April 2011, abstract 4295.
66 Lee FF, Foster CS: Pharmacotherapy of uveitis. Expert Opin Pharmacother 2010;11:1135–1146.
67 Rodriguez-Martinez S, Cancino-Diaz ME, Jimenez-Zamudio L, Garcia-Latorre E, Cancino-Diaz JC: TLRs and NODs mRNA expression pattern in healthy mouse eye. Br J Ophthalmol 2005;89:904–910.
68 Gupta D, Agarwal R, Aggarwal AN, Jindal SK: Molecular evidence for the role of mycobacteria in sarcoidosis: a meta-analysis. Eur Res J 2007;30:508–516.
69 Yanagihori H, Oyama N, Nakamura K, Mizuki N, Oguma K, Kaneko F: Role of IL-12B promoter polymorphism in Adamantiades-Behcet's disease susceptibility: an involvement of Th1 immunoreactivity against *Streptococcus sanguinis* antigen. J Invest Dermatol 2006;126:1534–1540.
70 Saari KM, Vilppula A, Lassus A, Leirisalo M, Saari R: Ocular inflammation in Reiter's disease after *Salmonella enteritis*. Am J Ophthalmol 1980;90:63–68.
71 Taurog JD, Richardson JA, Croft JT, et al: The germfree state prevents development of gut and joint inflammatory disease in HLA-B27 transgenic rats. J Exp Med 1994;180:2359–2364.
72 Chang JH, McCluskey PJ, Wakefield D: Toll-like receptors in ocular immunity and the immunopathogenesis of inflammatory eye disease. Br J Ophthalmol 2006;90:103–108.
73 Rosenbaum JT, Rosenzweig HL, Smith JR, Martin TM, Planck SR: Uveitis secondary to bacterial products. Ophthalmic Res 2008;40:165–168.
74 McGonagle D, Savic S, McDermott MF: The NLR network and the immunological disease continuum of adaptive and innate immune-mediated inflammation against self. Semin Immunopathol 2007;29:303–313.
75 Stojanov S, Kastner DL: Familial autoinflammatory diseases: genetics, pathogenesis and treatment. Curr Opin Rheumatol 2005;17:586–599.
76 Rosenzweig HL, Galster KT, Planck SR, Rosenbaum JT: NOD1 expression in the eye and functional contribution to IL-1beta-dependent ocular inflammation in mice. Invest Ophthalmol Vis Sci 2009;50:1746–1753.
77 Rosenzweig HL, Planck SR, Rosenbaum JT: NLRs in immune privileged sites. Curr Opin Pharmacol 2011;11:423–428.
78 Zhang H: Anti-IL-1beta therapies. Recent Pat DNA Gene Seq 2011;5:126–135.
79 Hoffman HM, Amar NJ, Cartwright RC, et al: Durability of response to rilonacept (IL-1 Trap) in a phase 3 study of patients with cryopyrin-associated periodic syndromes: Familial cold auto-inflammatory syndrome and Muckle-Wells syndrome; in Am Acad Allergy Asthma Immunol Meet, Philadelphia, March 2008.
80 Arcalyst Resource Center Patient Information Brochure. Tarrytown, Regeneron Pharmaceuticals, 2008.
81 Ilaris (canakinumab) package insert. East Hanover, Novartis Pharmaceutical Corp.
82 Kineret (anakinra) package insert. Thousand Oaks, Amgen.
83 Geiler J, McDermott MF: Gevokizumab, an anti-IL-1beta mAb for the potential treatment of type 1 and 2 diabetes, rheumatoid arthritis and cardiovascular disease. Curr Opin Mol Ther 2010;12:755–769.
84 Gül A, Artim Esen B, Solinger A, Giustino L, Tugal Tutkun I: Safe, rapid-onset, and sustained biological activity of il-1 beta regulating antibody XOMA 052 in resistant uveitis of Behçet's disease: preliminary results of a pilot trial. Ann Rheum Dis 2010; 69(Suppl 3):178.
85 Yoshimura T, Sonoda KH, Ohguro N, et al: Involvement of Th17 cells and the effect of anti-IL-6 therapy in autoimmune uveitis. Rheumatology (Oxford) 2009;48:347–354.
86 Haruta H, Ohguro N, Fujimoto M, et al: Blockade of interleukin-6 signaling suppresses not only th17 but also interphotoreceptor retinoid binding protein-specific Th1 by promoting regulatory T cells in experimental autoimmune uveoretinitis. Invest Ophthalmol Vis Sci 2011;52:3264–3271.
87 Hohki S, Ohguro N, Haruta H, et al: Blockade of interleukin-6 signaling suppresses experimental autoimmune uveoretinitis by the inhibition of inflammatory Th17 responses. Exp Eye Res 2010;91:162–170.
88 RoACTEMRA® (tocilizumab) summary of product characteristics. Roche, 2011.

89 Jones G, Sebba A, Gu J, et al: Comparison of tocilizumab monotherapy versus methotrexate monotherapy in patients with moderate to severe rheumatoid arthritis: the AMBITION study. Ann Rheum Dis 2010;69:88–96.
90 Smolen JS, Beaulieu A, Rubbert-Roth A, et al: Effect of interleukin-6 receptor inhibition with tocilizumab in patients with rheumatoid arthritis (OPTION study): a double-blind, placebo-controlled, randomised trial. Lancet 2008;371:987–997.
91 Nishimoto N, Yoshizaki K, Maeda K, et al: Toxicity, pharmacokinetics, and dose-finding study of repetitive treatment with the humanized anti-interleukin 6 receptor antibody MRA in rheumatoid arthritis. Phase I/II clinical study. J Rheumatol 2003;30:1426–1435.
92 Nishimoto N, Yoshizaki K, Miyasaka N, et al: Treatment of rheumatoid arthritis with humanized anti-interleukin-6 receptor antibody: a multicenter, double-blind, placebo-controlled trial. Arthritis Rheum 2004;50:1761–1769.
93 Nishimoto N, Miyasaka N, Yamamoto K, Kawai S, Takeuchi T, Azuma J: Long-term safety and efficacy of tocilizumab, an anti-IL-6 receptor monoclonal antibody, in monotherapy, in patients with rheumatoid arthritis (the STREAM study): evidence of safety and efficacy in a 5-year extension study. Ann Rheum Dis 2009;68:1580–1584.
94 Genovese MC, McKay JD, Nasonov EL, et al: Interleukin-6 receptor inhibition with tocilizumab reduces disease activity in rheumatoid arthritis with inadequate response to disease-modifying antirheumatic drugs: the tocilizumab in combination with traditional disease-modifying antirheumatic drug therapy study. Arthritis Rheum 2008;58:2968–2980.
95 Choy E: RADIATE: more treatment options for patients with an inadequate response to tumor necrosis factor antagonists. Nat Clin Pract Rheumatol 2009;5:66–67.
96 Bourlais CL, Acar L, Zia H, Sado PA, Needham T, Leverge R: Ophthalmic drug delivery systems – recent advances. Prog Retin Eye Res 1998;17:33–58.
97 Gurny R, Kaltsatos V, Deshpande AA, Zignani M, Percicot C, Baeyens V: Ocular drug delivery in veterinary medicine. Adv Drug Deliv Rev 1997;28: 335–361.
98 Diepold RW KJ, Himber J, Gurny R, Lee VHL, Robinson JR, et al: Comparison of different models for the testing of pilocarpine eyedrops using conventional eyedrops as a novel depot formulation (nanoparticles). Graefes Arch Clin Exp Ophthalmol 1989;227:188–193.
99 Zimmer AK CP, Saettone MF, Zerbe H, Kreuter J: Evaluation of pilocarpine-loaded albumin particles as controlled drug delivery systems for the eye. 2. Coadministration with Bioadhesive and Viscous Polymer. J Control Release 1995;33:31–46.
100 Vandervoort J, Ludwig A: Preparation and evaluation of drug-loaded gelatin nanoparticles for topical ophthalmic use. Eur J Pharm Biopharm 2004;57: 251–261.
101 Marchal-Heussler L FH, Devissaguet JP, Hoffman M, Maincent P: Colloidal drug delivery systems for the eye. A comparison of the efficacy of three different polymers: poly- isobutylcyanoacrylate, poly-lactic-coglycolic acid, poly-epsilon-caprolactone. Pharm Sci 1992;2:98–104.
102 Bourges J-L, Gautier SE, Delie F, et al: Ocular drug delivery targeting the retina and retinal pigment epithelium using polylactide nanoparticles. Invest Ophthalmol Vis Sci 2003;44:3562–3569.
103 Eljarrat-Binstock E, Pe'er J, Domb AJ: New techniques for drug delivery to the posterior eye segment. Pharm Res 2010;27:530–543.
104 Moritera T, Ogura Y, Yoshimura N, et al: Biodegradable microspheres containing adriamycin in the treatment of proliferative vitreoretinopathy. Invest Ophthalmol Vis Sci 1992;33:3125–130.
105 Guidetti B, Azema J, Malet-Martino M, Martino R: Delivery systems for the treatment of proliferative vitreoretinopathy: materials, devices and colloidal carriers. Curr Drug Deliv 2008;5:7–19.
106 Saishin Y, Silva RL, Saishin Y, et al: Periocular injection of microspheres containing PKC412 inhibits choroidal neovascularization in a porcine model. Invest Ophthalmol Vis Sci 2003;44:4989–4993.
107 Carrasquillo KG, Ricker JA, Rigas IK, Miller JW, Gragoudas ES, Adamis AP: Controlled delivery of the anti-VEGF aptamer EYE001 with poly(lactic-co-glycolic)acid microspheres. Invest Ophthalmol Vis Sci 2003;44:290–299.
108 Eljarrat-Binstock E, Domb AJ: A non-invasive ocular drug delivery. J Control Release 2006;110:479–489.
109 Kasting GB: Theoretical models for iontophoretic delivery. Adv Drug Deliv Rev 1992;9:177–199.
110 Pikal MJ: The role of electroosmotic flow in transdermal iontophoresis. Adv Drug Deliv Rev 2001;46: 281–305.
111 Molokhia SA, Jeong EK, Higuchi WI, Li SK: Examination of barriers and barrier alteration in transscleral iontophoresis. J Pharm Sci 2008;97: 831–844.

112 Behar-Cohen FF, Aouni A EI, Gautier S, et al: Transscleral Coulomb-controlled iontophoresis of methylprednisolone into the rabbit eye: influence of duration of treatment, current intensity and drug concentration on ocular tissue and fluid levels. Exp Eye Res 2002;74:51–59.
113 Sarraf D, Equi RA, Holland GN, Yoshizumi MO, Lee DA: Transscleral iontophoresis of foscarnet. Am J Ophthalmol 1993;115:748–754.
114 Chauvaud D, Behar-Cohen FF, Parel JM, Renard G: Transscleral Iontophoresis of cortcicosteoids: phase II clinical trial. Invest Ophthalmol Vis Sci 2000; 41:S79–S80.
115 Behar-Cohen F, Halhal M, Renard G, Bejjani RA: Corneal graft rejection and corticoid iontophoresis: 3 case reports. J Fr Ophtalmol 2003;26:391–395.
116 Behar-Cohen FF, Halhal M, BenEzra D, Chauvaud D, Renard G: Reversal of corneal graft rejection by iontophoresis of methylprednisolone. Invest Ophthalmol Vis Sci 2002;43:U504–U504.

Quan Dong Nguyen, MD, MSc
Diseases of the Retina and Vitreous, and Uveitis
Wilmer Eye Institute
Johns Hopkins University School of Medicine
600 North Wolfe Street, Maumenee 745
Baltimore, MD 21287 (USA)
E-Mail qnguyen4@jhmi.edu

Subject Index